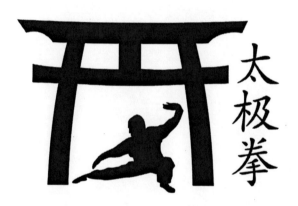

Phil Robinson Tai Chi

TAI CHI

THE WAY OF BALANCE IN AN UNBALANCED WORLD

A COMPLETE GUIDE TO TAI CHI AND HOW IT CAN STABILIZE YOU LIFE

PHIL ROBINSON

authorHOUSE®

AuthorHouse™
1663 Liberty Drive
Bloomington, IN 47403
www.authorhouse.com
Phone: 1-800-839-8640

First published by AuthorHouse 2/28/2011

ISBN: 978-1-4567-5114-2 (sc)
ISBN: 978-1-4567-5113-5 (e)

Library of Congress Control Number: 2011903304

Printed in the United States of America

THIS BOOK IS DEDICATED TO THE MEMORY OF:

KEN MCGUIRE

Sifu, 7th Degree Black Belt, Kenpo Karate

"He taught so many so much and died so soon"

DISCLAIMER

This book contains physical exercise that has its roots in the martial art of tai chi chuan.

As with any physical activity, extreme care, preparation and proper warm-up should be employed.

Many of these tai chi exercises are quite sophisticated and, as such, the oversight of a qualified tai chi master is necessary.

Due to the nature of these exercises, IT IS ESSENTIAL THAT A PHYSICIAN BE CONSULTED before engaging in these exercises.

Every possible effort has been made by the author to ensure the exercises are safe and effective. Therefore, the publisher and author are not responsible for any injury which may occur as a result of following the instructions written in this book.

SPECIAL ACKNOWLEDGEMENTS

I wish to thank and acknowledge all who have a desire to better their life by means of the use of tai chi principles. I acknowledge all of you who are trying to achieve balance in an unbalanced world.

This book has been a team effort:

Jerry Fuchs, "Fooksie" did the artwork and advised me.

Ziana de Bethune, Canadian author and tai chi student, who did what she could to help me.

Michael Connell did the editing.

Donna Robinson gave much advice and helped me remember.

Preston Sturgis helped me through my ignorance about computers and worked with formatting.

Mark Schmetzer, my webmaster, who formatted all the illustrations.

My students gave me the inspiration.

The biggest inspiration has been my student, Jeanne. At 82 years old, she has taught me more than I will ever teach her.

CONTENTS

1: SOME SPECIAL STUDENTS I HAVE KNOWN   1

     Jerry Fuchs   2

     Doug   4

     The Goat Keeper   6

     Jeanne   9

     Maggie   11

2: INTRODUCTION TO TAI CHI: ITS ORIGIN
AND BACKGROUND   15

3: START AT THE BEGINNING   23

     Tai Chi Styles   24

     Public Tai Chi   26

     Family Tai Chi   26

     How To Pick A School   27

     Know Yourself   28

     Establish A Planned Schedule   30

4: THIRTY MINUTES OF PARADISE   35

5: TAOIST INFLUENCE IN TAI CHI   45

     Verse 8: The Highest Good   50

     Verse 26: Seductions   52

     Verse 68: The Ethics Of War   53

     Verse 78: Appearance And Reality   54

     Verse 76: Let Yin Predominate Over Yang   56

6: THE CHI IN TAI CHI   59

     What Is Chi?   59

The Mind Directs The Chi, Therefore, You Must
Concentrate 64
Relax The Mind And Body 68
It Is Imperative To Breathe Properly 74
Put Your Mind, Body And Breath In Sync As One 77
Put It All Together With Tai Chi Moves 78
Simple, Isn't It? 79

7: MAINTAIN BALANCE AT ALL TIMES 81
Bio-Mechanical Balance 81
Physical Balance 85
Mental/Spiritual Balance 88
Yin /Yang......The Symbol Of True Balance 90
Yin Yang In Tai Chi 93

8: QIGONG, TAI CHI'S OLDER COUSIN 97

9: A FEW WORDS ABOUT TEACHING 105

10: THE TENS 113
Ten Benefits Of Tai Chi 113
Ten Ways To Ensure A Good Tai Chi Form 114
Ten Ways To Ensure A Good Tai Chi Workout 114
Ten Steps To Meditation 115
Ten Steps To Proper Breathing 116
Ten Words To Live By 116
Ten Stretches That Will Help 117
Ten Everyday Experiences Wherein Tai Chi Can
Assist 118
Ten Ways Tai Chi Principles Can Help A Marriage 119
Ten Ways To Train For Self Defense 122

11: NEAT STUFF THAT IS NICE TO KNOW 125
A Glossary Of Terms 125
Trees In Tai Chi, Qigong 128

The Negative Ion Advantage   129
Tai Chi Linage   131
Learning The Movements In The Form   131
Illustrations   138
    Illustrations for Learning the Form   138
    Linage Graph   152
    Yin/Yang Symbol   152

12: PARTING THOUGHTS   153

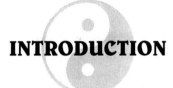

INTRODUCTION

Where were you in 1972? In 1972, President Nixon ré-opened trade with China for the first time since they became Communist in 1949. It is rather hard to imagine that in 1972 you could pick up anything in a store in this entire country and it did not say made in China. Each night for five days ABC news had a one hour special on China and Chinese culture.

Here we sat in our living rooms all across America and watched televisions that were complemented with rabbit ears. If you were rich, you had an antenna on top of your house, or if you lived in the Southern United States, also called "The South", your antenna was most likely nailed to a pine tree. Televisions with all the color quality of a Big Foot tape. So here we sat, an entire generation of Americans who knew nothing of China could now watch in our living room a world we had never seen before.

One evening, they had a program devoted to martial arts in China, tai chi being one of them. I sat with my mouth open in total amazement as I watched old men in their 70s and 80s tossing around young, strong men with no effort on their part. The narrator explained to us that tai chi was an ancient mystery and these very mature and overweight men were able to do these moves because of a chi force which Americans did not know existed.

I was 23 at the time. I was a young man with a wife and baby; a young man with an extensive background in boxing and karate (tang soo do); a young man whose life was about to change forever. By the time the program was over, I said, "I must learn tai chi. It is like nothing else." It took me three years to find a Chinese person willing to teach me. In 1975, I took my first class. My first instructor was Nancy Lee. She was the grandmother of a man I knew who managed a Chinese restaurant. She looked so thin and frail. I could pick her up and carry her on top of my shoulder and not even know she was there. However, as I learned later, she was thin but she was not frail. Her strength and stamina were amazing. She spoke no English and she had no desire to learn, either. Her attitude was, "You can learn Chinese if you want to speak to me." She did, however, learn two words in English after I became her student: "stupid boy." I heard that a lot. Since I was her only student, I knew it was directed at me.

That was how my life as a tai chi student began. Now, over 35 years have passed and, even though I became a Master in 1996, I still view myself as a student. I am still a student because I am still learning about tai chi. Tai chi unfolds throughout your whole life. The learning never ends. Here is an additional thought. I think you should be suspicious of any martial arts instructor who **insists** you call him Master. In the first place, we never master anything and in the second place, we should have only one Master and I am not him.

I truly hope you enjoy this book. My purpose in writing it is to help you understand more about the world of martial arts and the part tai chi plays in that world and the part it can play in your world.

If you learn something, if it helps you, if it makes you smile, then my job is done.

I wish to thank my teachers: Nancy Lee, Jim Hamilton, Lawrence Haung, Sharon Townsend, Ken McGuire, Soon Wong Bak, Mike Donaldson and David Glass. I am the sum total of these people and what I am as a martial artist, I owe to them.

I want to acknowledge my wife, Donna, my stepson, Chris, my children, Nicolle, Matt, Shane and Lacey and my grandchildren, Zachary, Dakota, Joshua and Bella; who all understand I am primarily a martial artist who also happens to be a husband, a father and a granddaddy.

1

SOME SPECIAL STUDENTS
I HAVE KNOWN

Back in the mid '80s, when my kids were in school, I came by to pick up my son who was in the 3rd grade. I met with the principle, Mr. Beaver, in the hallway and I noticed, as the children were walking by, he would speak to about one of every three and call them by name. "Hello, Sarah, see you tomorrow. See you in the morning, Kevin". And so it would go. I asked him, "Do you know everyone's name in this school?"He said, "No, just the real good ones and the real bad ones". That statement has stuck with me for more than 20 years now and it is amazing how well it applies to life and how well it fits the life of a martial arts instructor. In the 30 plus years I have taught, thousands have entered my class and, within the setting of the classroom, I have made my best friends and confronted my worst enemies. I am going to share with you a few of the best ones who have left a mark on my memory. Some of them changed the way I think about things and all inspired me. I am thinking their experience will inspire you, too.

JERRY FUCHS

Fuchs is German for fox and it is pronounced like you would pronounce books with the letter "f" instead of the letter "b". When I first saw his name on the student application I said, "Well, I see why you want to study martial arts. With a name like that, you probably get teased a lot." He laughed a silly boyish laugh and then told me he had just moved from New Jersey and was looking for a dojo where he could work out. He was a black belt in Ishin-Ryu. There was just something about him you just couldn't help but like. He looked like most people would imagine a German/American to look. He was tall, about 6'4", slim build, blue eyes, blonde hair, very disciplined and yet he always carried a winning smile. As it worked out, he learned tai chi at my school and he showed me Ishin-Ryu techniques. This man had a wealth of knowledge. He studied Japanese. He performed all his katas and techniques to the point they were a thing of beauty. The best all-around fighter I have ever seen….ever. In spite of his size and power, he was so kind and good to all. He gave so much to so many of my students and never once asked for a dime or any special treatment. As you might expect, with his Karate background, he learned the tai chi moves quickly. He worked as a commercial artist who was hired by a laser company and he designed many laser shows that were shown in Atlanta, Georgia and drew tourists from all over the United States. As an artist, he produced many of my ads and my tai chi logo. He even designed the front cover of this book. Again, he never once asked for a dime. He always refused money when it was offered.

In 1996, Jerry and I went to the Olympics in Atlanta to see the judo matches. He made friends with a Japanese family sitting in front of us and conversed with them in Japanese and took pictures of them with their camera. As it turned out, the man who won the Gold Metal was Japanese. His father was the man sitting in front of us that Jerry had befriended. All of a sudden, we were surrounded by news cameras from all over the world. Not only was this man the winner's father but a famous Judo champion himself. He insisted that his picture be taken with Jerry and me and that it would be in the Tokyo newspaper. I'm thinking, "Here we have Japanese, a German/American and a Scottish/American all hugging and smiling and getting along. It wasn't just us. It was people from all around the world, happy together. That's what the Olympics are all about. That is what Martial Arts are all about." As a Tai Chi master, I can go anywhere in the world and be embraced and trusted. I can cross any language barrier and receive respect from another tai chi artist. That is what Jerry Fuchs taught me that day. And, as always, he taught by example not by words. He was always the first to offer help, the first to offer friendship, the last to ask for anything.

In 1998, I received a phone call from Jerry. He was in the hospital. He had just been diagnosed with M.S. and was paralyzed from his chest down. I took in a deep breath, looked around as if to find someone to help me, swallowed hard, and fought back the tears. All the times he was strong for us, it was my turn to be strong for him. So I said, "Way to go Jerry, you don't screw up often, but when you do, you go all out", as I forced a nervous laugh. Then I told him, "Now it is time for you to dig down and fight. This is when you really use your tai chi, when you really use your karate. The spirit of the ancient warriors is in you represented by all your techniques. Use this to heal." He said, "Tell my wife to bring me the t-shirt you gave me. I am going to put it on and start to fight." And fight he did. I told you already he was a good fighter.

When he was released from the hospital, his wife brought him to see me at my school. He could walk some, but could not climb the steps without help. We worked all day on the tai chi healing techniques. We did "tree in winter"," the stork technique", "hug the tree", and "hold the lute" and others. He worked and worked and worked on these healing techniques. Not for a couple of days, but for years. Today, with the help of medical science, and the healing power of tai chi in the hands of a true martial artist, Jerry is doing fine. Some days are better others. But still, after twelve years fighting M.S., he shows no signs of giving up or slowing down. He came to my birthday party in 2003. I had martial arts friends from all over. There were seven different styles and three foreign countries represented at this party. As always, when we get together, we spar until we drop and then we start the party. That night, I turned 55. Jerry Fuchs kicked my butt as if he had never been sick a day in his life.

It is all too clear why I will always remember Jerry. It is all too clear what I learned from him. It is not what I taught him, but what he taught me. Jerry is one of the best examples of the healing power of tai chi you will ever find. It has been more than seven years since that birthday party and Sensei Jerry Fuchs, "Fooksie" is still well and happy.

DOUG

Doug and I have very little in common. He is young, I am old. He is a computer genius and loves computers, I can barely navigate through my computer and many times I think my computer would make a better boat anchor than a personal "do everything for me" tool that makes up most of my world.

He is raising children, mine are grown and gone. He drives a new high end luxury SUV. I drive a 14 year old pickup truck. Not much in common, you might say.

It has been said that, "politics make strange bedfellows". It can be said that "tai chi makes strange bedfellows" as well. Doug and I do have the tai chi in common, which is a unique bond that can only be understood if you study tai chi under a true master. Doug's main purpose for studying tai chi was stress reduction. Since I knew that up front, I centered his instruction around the stress reduction aspects of tai chi. You see, tai chi is all encompassing and people study tai chi for many different reasons: Stress reduction, balance, mental health, philosophy, self defense, muscle tone, flexibility, relief of arthritis pain, or just because it is something Chinese. These are a few reasons people take tai chi. There are many more and tai chi can do it all for you. As a tai chi instructor, one has to be able to fulfill the needs of the individual as well as the class.

As I said, Doug's interest in tai chi was stress reduction. This came in quite handy at a crossroads in his life. He works in corporate America where stress is a daily occurrence.

The day came where he had an opportunity to move up the ladder and out the building. He was going to interview for a new job with a different company .This meant more money and far better hours. One little catch about the interview, the man doing the interview was notorious for being loud, arrogant, and really intimidated people to the point where many left his office in tears and never finished the interview. Knowing this ahead of time, Doug practiced and practiced the stress reduction techniques that are the foundation of tai chi. He practiced right up to the time he entered the office for the interview. As he entered the office, he entered with the calm, confident air of an ancient warrior going into battle. From the very outset, the interviewer yelled at him and insulted him. This did not rattle Doug in the least. He remained calm and confident throughout. As the interview progressed, the calmer Doug remained, the calmer the interviewer became and, by the time the interview was over, the interviewer had abandoned his belligerent attitude and was friendly. Doug did get the job.

Did tai chi and its relaxation skills help Doug get this job? Well, yeah. I think I would be within the mark if I said he would not have been hired had it not been for the tai chi principles he practiced. The key word here is PRACTICED. He practiced regularly. What makes a good pitcher, a good quarterback, a good golfer, a good dancer, a good tai chi student, is practice. Doug is a good example of what practicing tai chi can do for you in your life.

THE GOAT KEEPER

I could never write a book or any thoughts about my students without saying a few words about the

Goat Keeper. OK, I will tell you how he received the name "Goat Keeper". His name is really Ray and he became a student of mine in 1994 and to this day is still a student. That is 16 years, as of now, about 112 in dog years. So let's rewind.

In 1992, I owned a school in downtown Stone Mountain, GA, right on Main Street. Stone Mountain was once a semi-rural small town that was complete with tin roofs, moonshine stills, dirt roads and everything else associated with the Old South. When I was growing up during the 1950s and '60s, I would walk to Stone Mountain from my house, climb the mountain, walk back to Atlanta and be home before dark. Even though it was only 12 miles east of Atlanta, it was like walking into an entirely different world. The people, the roads, the houses were all different from what I was used to in Atlanta. The City also bears the distinction of having the largest piece of exposed granite in the world. Oh yes, a great big rock. It is quite impressive, especially if you have traveled 400 miles with a car load of kids and empty McDonald's sacks to see it. This rock mountain has a base of 500 acres and is quite a climb to the top. In the 1920s it was owned by one person who thought it would be a great idea to carve a statue of some of the Confederate War Generals on the side of this mountain. The carving is larger than a football field. The carving project had several delays and when it was finally finished in 1973, Vice President Spiro Agnew came and dedicated it. Spiro Agnew and Confederate Generals... two great winners. Well, time marches on and by the time I opened my school in 1992, gone were the dirt roads and tin roofed houses and with it, much of the old way of thinking was gone, and had been replaced by more modern thinking. By then, Stone Mountain, Georgia had evolved into a tourist town and Main Street had been converted to a quaint village for tourists who come from all over to climb a big rock. My school was right on Main Street on the outskirts of the Village of Stone Mountain. It was right beside City Hall, which, in days gone by, was the train depot.

By 1992, 50,000 people drove down Main Street and right by my school every day. This was because all the cotton fields had been converted to subdivisions. When attendance would get low in the beginners class, I would take some white construction paper and a sharpie pen and write: "Tai Chi for Beginners, Class Now Forming" and I would place it in the window. That was all it took. Within a week, the class was full again.

In the summer of 1994, I placed that sign in the window. In comes a man who is bigger than most pro football players. He comes up to me and says, "I'm Ray. Are you the marketing genius with the sharpie pen?" So, he signs up.

As I said, MUCH of the old south was gone. Not all of it. Across the street from the school was a big old house that was converted into The Church of Old Time Christian Religion. Once, on a Monday and Tuesday evening, they carried signs in front of their church that informed everyone that "martial arts are evil and tai chi is from the Devil." I never thanked them for the free advertisement. That Wednesday night I addressed the class by saying that the church across the street is carrying signs that say tai chi is from the Devil. Could it be, Satan?

Upon hearing this, Ray says, "If tai chi is from the Devil, then I will be the Goat Keeper." And from that day forward, the name stuck. There has been at least 1,200 people come and go who never knew his name other than the Goat Keeper. And most never knew why he had such an unusual name.

It has been said that, once you learn of something that is really good, you will become either a monk or a missionary for the cause. In other words, once you learn tai chi, you will lock it up inside you and keep it to yourself (like a monk) or you will want to tell the world about your tai chi (like a missionary). Goat Keeper is definitely a missionary. His favorite expression is, "You should try tai chi. You will never sweat so much while moving so slow." [Sic]

Throughout the years, Goat Keeper has hit a few speed bumps. He has endured a divorce, a child who needed a kidney transplant, the death of his mother, and other ups and downs that many of us experience. Through all these things happening in his life he never once abandoned tai chi and never once missed a class and never once forgot to practice. He was a wine merchant, by trade, and would travel the world tasting and purchasing wine; a hard job, indeed. He was learning the "cloud hands" part of the form and had to go to Paris. There he was, early in the morning, practicing "cloud hands" on the sidewalks of Paris. He did get a few stares, but when he arrived home, he knew "cloud hands".

What I learned from Goat Keeper could be summed up in one word: consistency. Rich or poor, happy or sad, sick or well, Goat Keeper has always been consistent in his practice.

In 2005, we had a tea ceremony and Goat Keeper was promoted to Sifu, or instructor. He has retired now, and no longer works full-time and like all of us, is getting older. Every Sunday morning at 8:30, you will see him in the park along the Etowah River in Cartersville, GA performing Yang Tai Chi with the same zeal he had as a beginner.

JEANNE

At the time of the writing of this book, Jeanne has been a student of mine for about a year. Even though she has been a student for a short time, she has left a mark on the memory of many, myself included. She is tall, thin, blue eyes quite classy and good looking. Oh, and did I mention, she is 82 years old.

It seems she gets along better with people in their 50s and 60s than she does people her age. All her friends are much younger than she. This is because she thinks and acts like a young person. Once a month, at one of the places I teach, there is a free luncheon for seniors and she always seems to be uncomfortable around these older people. She just does not fit in. Such a spark of life she brings to the class each week! And Jeanne is so funny, she will say just about anything.

I remember when she first started, she had been taking tai chi about three weeks, I could not help but notice that she was catching on to the moves and postures so easily, especially for someone her age. Often, someone who has never taken tai chi before but has a background in dance or karate will catch on faster and will look better with their moves than someone who has never done anything where mental and physical co-ordination are required. So I asked her, "Hey, Jeanne, have you ever done any dancing?" She smiled and said, "Only on table tops". That was the last thing I expected to hear from an 82- year-old woman and, no doubt one of the funniest. That's Jeanne. You can't be around her for ten minutes and you are laughing at something she has said or done.

The main reason for her starting the class was not for her health or to attain more energy. She simply wanted to learn it and do the moves right and she decided I was the one who could teach her.

After about a month into it and, as the postures became more complicated, she began to have difficulty with her balance. Improving your balance is so important. Over one third of the people over 65 become disabled or die due to complications from falls. There is documented evidence that proves tai chi can drastically improve the balance in the over 65 group and has great success in fall prevention. With all this in mind, I set out to help Jeanne with her balance. When she began to realize it was not going to be easy and it was going to take some time, she did not give up, she did not complain, she did not make excuses and quit. Instead she started to take private lessons, she started coming to three classes a week instead of just one, and she practiced every day, early in the morning. Every class, at least once she would say, "I am going to get this, and when I do, it's going to be right."

It is my joy to tell you that in nine month's time, her balance has improved by 60%. When she started she could stand on one foot for five seconds. Now she has no trouble standing for fifteen or twenty seconds. Perhaps that doesn't sound like much. If you believe this is easy, get a timer and set it for twenty seconds and stand on one leg and see how it easy and fun it is. I am willing to bet that would be one of the longest twenty seconds you will ever experience. Now, throw into the mix, she happens to be 82.

Here is one lady who has taken hold of her life and has made herself stronger, smarter and better balanced than she was a year ago. Was it tai chi that gave to her all this new health, energy and balance in her life? I like to think it was her youthful attitude, her sense of humor, the ability to laugh at herself and her dogged determination to better herself that made the difference. Tai chi just happened to be there and was the vehicle God chose to keep this wonderful lady healthy. It has been my extreme pleasure to guide her through these tai chi teachings.

MAGGIE

The first day she entered my school, she was a quiet, shy young lady who was 15 years old. When she talked to you, she would look down at her shoes and not look at you in the face. She was quite pretty. She had long straight auburn / reddish hair with dark eyes and an olive complexion. She was a mix of Native American and Irish, which is not uncommon in the South. It occurred to me she was a classic example of someone who had a complete lack of self-confidence.

As it turned out, martial arts training is just what she needed. She became stronger and more muscular, her countenance was improving and her concentration skills had greatly increased. I began to notice that as her martial arts improved and as she mastered more and more difficult postures and moves, her self-confidence was increasing in direct proportion with her progress in class.

By the time she left the school, she transformed herself from a mousy little girl who was constantly looking down to a strong willed woman who looked you straight in the eye.

You see, it's like this. There is only one way to gain more confidence, and that is to successfully complete a difficult task. If you never reach out and learn a new language or never reach out and learn to play a musical instrument, or never reach out and master a tai chi form or a karate kata you will never have the confidence you could have had. And you know what that means? It means you will never have the success you could have had. I believe that is why you seldom see a tai chi master or a true karate master who is a failure in life or one who has money problems. The confidence and discipline that the practice of tai chi produces spills over into your daily life and makes you a better person.

This thought was made manifest in Maggie's case. Later, she became a restaurant manager in Atlanta, and is a successful, well educated woman. Do you think she would have reached the level of success she has reached had she never studied tai chi and the martial arts and never gained confidence? You tell me.

In conclusion, it has been said that the best way to learn something is to have to teach it. I agree. I would like to add to that not only do you learn the material you are teaching in tai chi but you learn so much more about life and how tai chi principles can improve life.

I have learned from my students that tai chi has an enormous healing power. I have seen tumors disappear, I have seen cancer go away, and I have seen MS stay in remission. I have seen people remain calm during circumstances that were quite stressful and could drive some insane. I have seen the weak made powerful and the arrogant made humble. I have seen total dedication to tai chi and total apathy toward tai chi.

If there is one thing I have learned from my students, it would be this: Tai chi is an ancient martial art based on the ancient wisdom of Taoist philosophy. Nothing more, nothing less. The enormous benefits that come from tai chi are a direct result of the effort you put into it.

I have had students quit tai chi because they wanted to work on Christmas lights. On the other hand, I have seen people so sick they could hardly stand up practice every day. Tai chi is not a magical path to true enlightenment and absolute healing. Tai chi is what you make of it. And, as always, anything worthwhile requires hard work.

If you do not read another chapter in this book, that is OK. You have already read the chapter that matters most. You were able to meet five of my students. Would you please do me a favor? Put down this book for a minute and ponder Jerry, Maggie, Doug, Jeanne, and Goat Keeper and think of how tai chi has affected their lives and how you can learn from their examples. If you would like to be more like these five, pick the book back up, because it is going to get interesting.

2

INTRODUCTION TO TAI CHI: ITS ORIGIN AND BACKGROUND

When I was a small boy, around ten or twelve years old, my friend and I would take the bus to downtown Atlanta and go to the movies on Saturday. We never once thought about checking a theater schedule. We would arrive, enter the theater, sit down and start watching the movie. Sometimes, it was already half over. It didn't matter. When the movie ended, we would sit there and watch it from the beginning. When we came to the part that was showing when we entered the theater, I would say to my friend, "This is where we came in. Do you want to stay and watch it over or leave now?"

Tai chi is a little like that. The underlying principles of tai chi date back to the earliest of times in recorded history. There are even some tai chi postures discovered written on tortoise shells that date back to 1000 BC. Where we come in on tai chi is in the 1700s. A General Chen retired from military life and decided to put together 105 of his favorite moves on the battle field. These moves had stood the test of time and had been perfected and honed and sharpened by the lives of thousands of ancient warriors. It was his intention to open a school in his village and teach these 105 moves for some extra money since now he was a poor farmer and the military did not have much of a pension plan in the 1700's. He named his new venture "Chen t'ai jing chuan" In English, it would say, "The supreme ultimate way of fighting (boxing) according to Chen". What a great idea! He designed a pattern of 105 moves where one moved into the other without stopping. It looked like a fast, jerky dance that didn't stop for 20 minutes. There was no defense against these moves. Most were deadly and quick. You became an unstoppable force. There was one small problem. His tai chi business was a financial disaster. He would come home to his wife each night and she would say, "How did it go today?" And he answered, "Horrible, I made no money today, no one wants my tai jing chuan and it is the best there is in all of China." His wife was sitting at their homemade table in the middle of a dirt floor drinking tea and she looks up from her tea cup and says, "Well, that's because only the old people in the village have money. Maybe you should slow these moves down so the older ones can join in. It would be good exercise for them and you could make some money." General Chen's eyes grew large and he said, "That's the stupidest thing I ever heard! I will never do that and compromise my t'ai jing chuan."

One day a young Taoist priest entered Chen's class, having gone through some difficulty being accepted because he was an outsider and not a member of the Chen linage. His name was Yang (pronounced Young). Does that sound familiar? It will. Being a Taoist priest, Yang had a background in deep spiritual meditation, the healing power of herbs, a philosophy based on the Tao Te Ch'ing, an ancient holy book. He knew the importance of balance in life from a mental, physical and spiritual standpoint. He even knew how to balance a meal properly to get the most nutrition and the least stress on the body. Have you ever eaten a Chinese meal and been hungry in two hours? It is supposed to be that way. Chinese meals are balanced by Taoist principles of yin /yang and go through your system quickly. This is not because they are empty calories, but because this food is balanced in your system. Yang knew all this and, by the way, he also knew how to fight….some. All priests did because they were constantly traveling from village to village and were subject to robbery and attacks. In the 1700's, a Taoist priest was a holy man, a doctor, a scholar, a nutritionist and a scientist with knowledge of chemistry all rolled into one. It amazes me that a Taoist Priest was all this and knew all this before we ever made a Constitution and formed this country.

So, as I said, Yang enters Chen's school and he works hard and becomes his star pupil. He can defeat anyone in the school, anyone in the village. Chen really likes this guy. He is smart, quick and very intelligent. One day Yang and Chen were talking and Yang says, "You know, Chen, if we slowed these moves down, the older people could join in class too, and they would benefit from the exercise." General Chen says, "I told my wife a long time ago I would never do that. I am a warrior and I shall die a warrior." So Yang says, "Well, if it is all the same to you, I would like to start my own style of t'ai jing chuan, perhaps in my home village." Chen says, "Well, good-bye. But it will never work."

So Yang sets out to make a martial art style that maintains balance at all times. You know how to fight, but you know how to avoid a fight. You know how to train hard, but you also know how to stretch and relax. You know how to anticipate a move and you know not to telegraph your move. You know for every push there is a pull, for every strike there is a block, for every kick there is a ward off. Yang chose the Yin/Yang symbol to symbolize his style because it represents total balance.

Guess what. He slowed down the moves for the older ones in the village. Now, as I said, this is where we come in on it. The beauty and magic of tai chi began to unfold as the moves were slowed down and modified for the older ones. The first thing Yang noticed was their complexions became better. Their cheeks became rosy and they felt better and looked better. They even had better balance. Why?

Yang, being a Taoist priest, had an inquisitive mind and the education to satisfy this curiosity. With research, he discovered when the moves are slow and your breath is in sync with your moves, it creates an abundant amount of internal energy called "chi". In connection with the tai jing chuan moves, this chi energy can now be directed throughout the body and used for healing and healthy energy. They now had rosy cheeks because this Yang style increased the blood circulation. Now, the slow moves, the body, the breath, the blood flow and the mind are all as one. Why were these older ones better balanced? Because it had as its foundation a martial art. In ancient days when fighting hand to hand, what would happen to you if you lost your balance on the battle field and fell to the ground? Do you think you would survive this fall? I really doubt the enemy would help you get up. General Chen put in his postures moves that were designed to give you a strong sense of balance at all times. So, you can say better balance is a byproduct of the martial art of t'ai jing chuan.

So Yang, with the help of some of his Taoist relatives, namely sons, grandsons and nephews, introduced a well balanced style of martial art for everyone young and old. It would protect you from evil thoughts through philosophy. It would protect you from illness by means of nutrition and chi force. It would protect you from weakness through discipline and exercise. It would protect you from any attacker with its superior martial art skills.

Yang had just what he wanted. He founded a balanced martial art that encompassed the entire spiritual, physical, emotional and mental aspects of the human being. He emphasized health, healing and relaxation over fighting. It was the chi force that was all important, not fighting.

Since the development of your personal chi was emphasized, he changed the name from t'ai jing chuan (supreme fighting) to t'ai chi chuan (supreme, ultimate energy). Since his name was Yang, he called it Yang T'ai Chi.

Since the days of Benjamin Franklin and Paul Revere, not much has changed in tai chi. From the Chen style, Yang, Sun, Wu and Hao (Han-Wu) styles branched off and created their own little world. To this day, pure traditional Chen Tai Chi is still a fast paced powerful style full of jerky moves, and fighting skills are on top of the list. Yang is still the most balanced and the most popular in the United States and throughout in the world, for that matter.

Here is an easy way to tell what you are looking for. Generally speaking, if the instructor claims he/she teaches tai chi, it is usually an exercise program that you will find at a fitness or recreation center. If the instructor claims to teach tai chi **chuan**, then, it is usually the entire spectrum of tai chi: exercise, meditation, self-defense, philosophy, etc. A brief word of caution: Be wise in selecting an instructor. There are many weekend wonders that really are quite uneducated in tai chi. I even saw someone teaching a class who had the "T'ai Chi For Dummies" book opened in front of them as they taught.

Clearly, much in the world has changed since the days of Chen. Legend has it he died a pauper on his farm. Little did he know he lit a torch that set the entire world ablaze.

What I have told you so far tells you in some detail the

origin of tai chi. I am sure you are smart enough to know there is far more to it than what I have mentioned. Also, I am sure you are smart enough to realize that part of what I mentioned was just a parable to prove a point. This is often called legend. In other words, I am not sure if Chen had a dirt floor in his house, but I am sure he was among the greatest martial artists who ever lived. At least we now know enough to understand that when we practice tai chi, we are participating in a past that is rich in knowledge and tradition.

As for the history of tai chi, I have decided not to bog you down with all the details of its history. It can get quite complicated and involved because so many families are involved at so many time periods. However, I did enter a spider graph at the back of the book that depicts all the family lines that were the founders of various tai chi styles and divisions. If you take tai chi, perhaps you can spend an hour or so and trace your style back to one of these original families. If that is what you like to do, that is fine. The bookshelves are full of tai chi books that spend half of their chapters discussing families with a linage that is complicated and contains somewhat of an ambiguous history. I don't think we need another one.

As far as the history of tai chi goes, know this: When you participate in tai chi, you participate in an ancient civilization that thought nothing of starting a building project that would last 1,000 years. It is a culture that has over 35,000 characters in its alphabet. It takes a lifetime to learn, and another lifetime to perfect. The culture has a long history of having a passion for education, enjoying complicated studies and makes everyday routines into works of art. When you participate in tai chi, you are literally "walking the way of ancient warriors". You are participating in an activity that was once made illegal throughout China and other regions and tai chi masters were tortured and killed. As recently as

1980, tai chi instructors were killed in Afghanistan by the Soviet Russians. (During Soviet Russia's occupation, there was a death penalty for practicing and/or teaching any style of martial art.) You will be participating in a culture that had a cure for pain and many major diseases while Europe was still in the dark ages. Yes, tai chi sprang from this history. It should come as no surprise that tai chi takes time and patience to learn, and a lifetime to master.

Speaking of mastering tai chi, the next chapter deals with some thoughts on how to do just that. To master tai chi, you must start at the beginning.

3

START AT THE BEGINNING

We have never met and I don't know you. I do know this: you must have some interest in tai chi. Otherwise, you would not be reading this book. You may be a very nice person who wants to better yourself and tai chi may be the way. You may be getting a little older and no longer want to run marathons and do step aerobics and you are looking for a low impact way to stay in shape. You may think tai chi can melt away your stress and help you live healthier and longer.

My thoughts in this book are directed to those who want to study tai chi, but get a little confused when they view a DVD or read a book about it. I am going to guide you through the maze that will result in your life becoming better as a result of being a student of tai chi. As I stated, we must start at the beginning.

The beginning can be divided into four different categories: 1. Have a basic knowledge of tai chi styles, so you will know what to look for when picking a school. 2. How to choose the right school. 3. Know yourself and know what you want to gain from the study of tai chi. 4. Once you have selected a style and a school, develop a scheduled program.

TAI CHI STYLES

I view styles of tai chi the same way I view religions of the world. There are so many religions with such differing philosophies, but they all have a common ground. That common ground is that people benefit from the practice of the principles contained in that religion which are usually written in a holy book that is as old as dirt. Regardless of the religion, you benefit. It is up to you to find a religion that best suits your personality. The same principle applies to tai chi. There are many different styles and types of tai chi and regardless of which style you study, you will benefit. It is up to you to find the one that best suits your personality.

CHEN STYLE:

Chen is the original tai chi, the granddaddy of them all. It is authentic, traditional and very Chinese. It was founded by Chen Chang Xing in the 1700's. Its characteristics are low stances with slow flowing moves that will suddenly explode into a violent jerky technique. It emphasizes physical fitness and fighting skills. In my opinion, in its pure form, it is not for the elderly or the out of shape.

YANG STYLE:

Yang tai chi is the most popular throughout the world. It is less than one generation newer than Chen style. As stated earlier, Yang style has a more balanced approach to life. Its characteristics are slow moving postures that are soft and flowing with no stress to the joints. It can be performed from either a low stance or a high stance. The self defense moves are very effective and easy to learn.

WU STYLE:

Wu style was founded in the mid 1800's by Wu Yu-Xiang, who was a previous student of the Yang style.

The stances are narrow and high. The hand postures contain many movements of large circles.

The moves are slow and harmonious. The self defense applications differ from Yang in that they contain mostly joint locks, throws and submission holds. It appears the self defense may have come from a source or style other than pure tai chi. In the United States, it seems that Wu style has evolved, for the most part, into a healthy exercise.

SUN STYLE:

Sun tai chi is the baby of the bunch. It was founded by Sun Lu Tang in the early 1900's, and is a hybrid of three different styles. It is not uncommon in the world of martial arts to take something you like from another style and add it to your style, while at the same time removing something from your original style that doesn't work for you. Martial Arts legend Bruce Lee did this constantly. Those who adhere to this practice say, "This new style is better and stronger than old tradition." Critics will say, "All they did is water down a style that was already perfect. They changed it because it was too difficult for them to learn." This controversy will go on forever. Sun is a good exercise, especially for the elderly or those with medical issues. Be advised that Sun tai chi has been modified many times, especially recently.

HAO (Han- Wu) STYLE:

You seldom hear of Hao outside of China and it is difficult to find out anything about Hao past the 1930's. It appears to be a spinoff of the Yang style as it contains the slow harmonious moves.

PUBLIC TAI CHI

These styles are referred to in China as "public tai chi". Meaning, tai chi that has a standardized curriculum and you can buy a book about it and study it at home. A style that you can take anywhere in China and the postures be the same. Public tai chi is what is taught in schools throughout China and the rest of the world. There is nothing wrong with public tai chi. About the only ones who find something wrong with it are people who do family tai chi.

FAMILY TAI CHI

There are at least 10,000 different styles of "family tai chi". Family tai chi is just that. It is tai chi that has stayed within the confines of a particular family for many generations, often kept a secret from outsiders. Kung Fu is the same way. So are moonshine formulas and fried chicken recipes in the South. All family tai chi has its roots in one of the four major styles, especially the first two. More often than not, there is a minor difference such as a hand position or angle of a posture. I have personally seen a family-based school break up and dissolve because of a dispute over the position of a single finger in one posture.

To share with you my experience in my 21 years as a student, I spent 14 years practicing family tai chi that had its roots in Yang. I spent 7 years studying public tai chi, Yang style. In the 14 years, I spent 5 years in Chen and the whole 14 years in Yang. There was a 5 year span where I studied two styles at the same time. As far as teaching in a commercial school goes, public tai chi was better for me simply because I could buy books and refer to them when I was not in class. My students could buy these books and refer to them at home (before the days of computer generated DVD's). Another thing I liked about public tai chi can be summed up in the following experience: At my school in Stone Mountain, GA, a man from California came through the door and wanted information about our tai chi. I told him our style and he said, "That's my style, too. Could we do Yang 24 together?" So we did, and it was identical. Here we are, almost 3,000 miles apart, 20 years difference in our ages, and our postures are identical. That's what I like about public tai chi. What I do is I start everyone in public tai chi and as they advance and show a desire to learn the deeper things, they transfer to the advanced class where family tai chi is taught. Here is where they can learn healing, herbs, diet, philosophy, and self defense applications. This is what I mean when I say "the deeper things".

So, here we have a brief synopsis of the styles tai chi has to offer. Now it is time to pick a style that best suits your personality. Next, find a school that teaches that style.

HOW TO PICK A SCHOOL

There are two and only two requirements for a school. 1. It needs to be close to home, no more than a 30 minute drive. 2. After the first 10 minutes you should feel comfortable and right at home. Since your tai chi class may continue for years, it is important to be as close to home as possible. It seems long trips to class do a lot to sap your joy. I am a big fan of trusting my feelings. If it feels right, do it. If it does not, then leave. Remember, this is not soccer where the season ends in 14 weeks or so. This should be a long-term commitment. You must feel comfortable with your instructor and at the same time be aware of his/her qualifications. If he looks about 22 and tells you he is a master and a linage holder, leave tire marks in the parking lot.

KNOW YOURSELF

Always, when a new student enters my school, the first question I ask is, "What do you want to gain by taking tai chi?" I have heard answers that range from, "I want them to stop killing the whales." to, "I would like to be able to beat up everyone on my softball team." This is true. I have actually had these answers. Most, however, want to participate in an exercise program that is good for them and reduce stress.

As a worksheet, I am going to list fifteen benefits tai chi offers and you check with a pencil five of these benefits you would like to enjoy the most:

1. Self defense, fighting skills
2. Greater flexibility
3. Lose weight
4. Stronger, firmer muscles
5. Better balance
6. More energy
7. Lower blood pressure
8. Stress release, relaxation
9. Learn meditation skills
10. Improve concentration
11. Pain control
12. Healing past physical injuries
13. Healing emotional scars
14. Acquire a healthy, happy attitude
15. Make them stop killing the whales

Of the five benefits you picked, if three or more of them were in the first seven on the list, then you are predominately a physical person and probably under 50 years old or at least act like you are. This being the case, you should consider a school that teaches everything from the moves to the self defense applications. If three or more that you checked were in benefits numbered 8 through 14, you are more of a spiritual person and a school that does not offer fighting skills would be fine for you. If you checked number 15, you are a flake and tai chi offers no hope for you. Maybe you should just go back to watching Animal Planet.

Take the five benefits you checked and ask the instructor how much time he spends on these benefits.

For example, ask: I need better flexibility, how much time is spent on stretching? How often do you do exercises that will improve my concentration? I am so forgetful. I have an old shoulder injury, can tai chi help? And so forth. Once you understand better what you want from tai chi, it will be easier for you to decide on your school.

You may be perfectly happy going to a recreation center or a church basement and taking tai chi from someone who did a weekend workshop and paid their money and received their very own "instructor's certificate". Here is where you will do some basic, often modified postures and do them week after week until this "certified" instructor goes to another seminar. On the other hand, you may want the real thing. You may want to learn tai chi the same way it was taught hundreds of years ago. You may want to learn all aspects of tai chi: health, healing, relaxation, self defense applications, philosophy and the spiritual side as well. Either way is fine, you will benefit either way. Just don't make the mistake of thinking someone who attended some seminars and have been around tai chi for five years or less can give you the real thing. That would be like asking someone who can sing happy birthday to conduct a symphony.

I want to share with you one final word about finding a school, a word that might surprise you. More often than not, a school will find you. If you are a true seeker of tai chi and if you look and ask around, you may be quite surprised how quickly one will turn up. I can't count the times someone has told me, "I have always wanted to take tai chi and I was driving home tonight and saw your sign on the road. And it's a funny thing, I never go home this way, but tonight I did." I even had a woman call me who cleaned offices at night and happened to pick up a newspaper on a table in the break room and before she threw it away, she saw my ad and called me right then.

So now we know how to pick a school and a style that suits our personality. Next, at the beginning, we need to establish a planned schedule.

ESTABLISH A PLANNED SCHEDULE

In the words of Billy Crystal, "A woman needs a reason to make love; all a man needs is a place." For your practice of tai chi, you need a place.

When you choose your place for practice, choose a place outside and inside. Outside is better because you will find there is far more energy outside. In meditation and in meditative postures you can draw in energy from the ground and trees around you, which helps in your flow of chi, which helps the body and soul. I have found it difficult to increase my chi inside while trying to draw energy from a nylon carpet. The absolute best case scenario is to practice your tai chi early in the morning, bare footed on grass that still has morning dew. This is where you can come in to harmony with your body, your soul, your mind, your internal feelings and nature as God planned it all at once. Outside also gives you a different perspective on things. You feel small and yet an important part of something bigger. If handled properly, the practice of tai chi outside can be a great exercise and a unique spiritual experience as well. Maybe that is why in China you see so many practicing their tai chi in the parks.

Besides, have you ever seen the houses they live in? Whoa!!! A little too small for tai chi.

You need to choose a place inside as well. Clearly, you can't be outside all the time and there are times you would rather be cool in the summer, warm in the winter and dry when it rains. When choosing a place inside, be sure it is quiet and roomy. It is a good thing to have a room with windows that can both let in sunlight and fresh air. Inside, if at all possible, you should be barefooted. While shoes can offer extra support and may give a beginner help with balance, being barefooted will help strengthen the muscles in your feet and will enable you to see your foot position while learning your postures. This is a special announcement: IF YOU ARE WEARING ORTHAPEDIC SHOES OR SPECIAL TENNIS SHOES FOR SUPPORT, DON'T TAKE THEM OFF. YOUR DOCTOR WILL NOT LIKE IT. YOU MAY FALL. The idea of going bare footed is a suggestion, not a command. Like anything else that involves physical movement, approach tai chi with a cautious and careful mind.

A very important key to choosing your place for practice is to practice in the same place each time, facing the same direction each time. Some experts say to start facing south. I do not agree. Just pick a direction and stick with it. In addition to being the same place, it should be the same time of day if possible. I will explain why a little later.

After picking a time and place, you should choose proper attire. Yes, proper attire. Choose comfortable, loose fitting clothes, flat shoes if you wear shoes. Many like to wear a t-shirt and sweat pants. I always wear a white t-shirt and black kung fu pants. You should buy a t-shirt that says tai chi on it. There are numerous places on the internet that will sell you a tai chi t-shirt. They usually cost 12.00 to 25.00. If you are attending a large commercial school, they many even have one for you.

You have now created your very own tai chi uniform. This uniform separates your tai chi from everything else going on in your life and when you put on this uniform you are mentally divorcing all your problems, thoughts, worries, medical issues and are completely focused on tai chi only. You should wear this uniform you created each time you practice at home, each time you attend class.

Do you see a pattern forming here? You practice in the same place, facing the same direction, the same time of day, in the same clothes while doing the same moves. It is called a consistent routine.

To this day, Buddhist Monks get up the same time every day and the first thing they do is go outside and rake sand in a box that is about 12 inches high and 6 feet square. They will rake north and south, east and west, draw circles, whatever. Then they give the rake to the Monk behind him in line and he does the same thing. Then it is breakfast. Why rake the sand? That is because it establishes a consistent routine. It is part of their training and discipline.

Do your utmost to be consistent. Which baseball player will make the most money: the one who hits a home run once in a while or a player who will consistently hit twenty five home runs year after year after year?

Picture in your mind a courtyard in an ancient Buddhist Temple in China today. Now picture in your mind twenty Buddhist Monks practicing their kung fu moves after breakfast in this courtyard. When was the last time you saw these Monks practicing in the courtyard and one was wearing cut off blue jeans and a tank top, another wearing baggie jeans with his plaid underwear showing and a baseball cap on backwards and another wearing sweat pants with holes in the thigh area and a t-shirt that says, "Party Till You Puke"?

Do you find that hard to imagine? I hope so. I really do not wish to be too hard on you here. But please remember this: You are honored to participate in a health and exercise program that reflects a culture that is thousands of years old. It is a culture that established a life of consistency. We demonstrate respect for this culture by being consistent in our training and dress. I promise you this consistent discipline will affect your daily life and make you a better person. Not to mention, it is the only way to master tai chi.

If you believe what I have told you in this chapter about consistent practice and consistent dress is stupid and is only so much bull feathers, that is no problem. You go right ahead and wear whatever you want, practice when you feel like it, and do it in all kinds of different places. Then check back with me in a year or so and let me know how your tai chi is working out for you.

If you have come this far, you should enjoy the next chapter. We are going to discuss thirty minutes of paradise.

4

THIRTY MINUTES OF PARADISE

For many of us, we are surrounded by things that cause us stress. Each new generation that springs forth, brings with it a new special kind of stress that is added on to the stress we already have in this world. All the inventions we have at our fingertips designed to save us time: the microwave oven, washer and dryer, air travel, the computer, instant this and instant that, super highway systems, the internet, cell phones, fax machines. All these things we have today that two generations ago no one had. In spite of having all these new inventions, the man who lived in 1910 on a farm with eight children had more time and far less stress than the man in 2010 who works in corporate America, has one child and every modern convenience at his beck and call. And these modern inventions that are designed to make life easier seem just to complicate life further and add to the stress in our life.

We have computer viruses, meltdowns, gridlocks on the expressway, spikes in our electrical system, inflation, higher taxes, unemployment, incurable diseases, teenage pregnancy, oil spills, air pollution, loud noise, violent crime, illegal drugs in every city, drive-by shootings, directions in four languages and not to mention, the threat of terrorist attacks at any minute, anywhere in our country. Have a nice day.

As the stress level increases, people are turning to ways to eliminate the stress in their lives by turning to alcohol, illegal drugs, prescription drugs and expensive counseling which more often than not, add to the stress they already have.

When it comes to stress release, there are two things that come to mind: 1.The example of my grandfather. 2. The thirty minutes of paradise that tai chi can offer.

First, my grandfather: He never borrowed money for anything except a house and a car. When he bought a car, he always kept it three years after it was paid for. He saved half the car payment money for a down payment on his next car and the other half he used to fix his old car that was paid for. He owned two pair of shoes, one for Sunday and one for work. He refused to accept credit cards. He called them plastic poverty. He never cheated on his wife and never drank himself silly. So, he created for himself a simple life that had little stress. What you can learn from this example is the amount of stress in your life is directly proportional to the decisions you make. We are all a product of our own decisions. The clothes we wear, the car we drive, the money we have, the husband or wife we have, even the fact that you are reading these words are all a direct result of decisions you have made. My grandfather did not live a stress free life. He was a City of Atlanta detective, owned a dog kennel on the side and he raised me. When he did get in stressful situations he would go in the yard, look at the trees and just take a deep breath. Once I asked him what he was doing and he told me he was just thinking of the mountains and streams he had left behind in his homeland. And then he said, "I just needed a little bit of paradise to help me get through this mess."

He died when I was 21 and forty years later, I still miss him. When I was 25, I discovered tai chi and discovered it had similar stress reduction and relaxation principles about it that were similar to my grandfather's. However, it is no big surprise that the relaxation and stress reduction techniques are a little more complicated in tai chi than they were in grandfather's yard. However, they both created paradise.

The number one reason people have come to me for tai chi instruction is for relaxation and stress reduction. My favorite part of tai chi is the total sense of calm you feel when you practice it properly. You can take your tai chi anywhere and use your thirty minutes of paradise to completely relax. You can take it to the beach or to a motel room when you travel. You can take it with you in the car when you are stuck in traffic. Anywhere, anytime you can use your thirty minutes of paradise to make you feel better. I once had a student who stayed with me for a little more than two years and he never progressed past the third posture, called brush the knee. He was not lazy, nor was he stupid or in any way physically challenged. He was happy staying right where he was after two years of practice doing the postures it takes most three to six weeks to learn. He told me, "I come here for the feeling I get. I get a special feeling of calmness here that I don't get anywhere else. For me, it is not the learning and advancement, it is the feeling." Now, why didn't I think of that? Tai chi is all about the feeling! Tai chi is all about creating your very own thirty minutes of paradise. All you need is a space about four by six feet. So let's get started.

First, we will work on breathing. Get as comfortable as possible. Many like to recline in an overstuffed recliner, some lie on the floor, it does not matter just get comfortable.

It must be quiet and undisturbed. Now, on a count of four, breathe in your nose: in one, two, three, four. Now, breathe out your mouth on a count of four: out one, two three, four. If you place the tip of your tongue to the roof of your mouth, it will benefit you. Placing the tongue to the roof of the mouth helps prevent your mouth from getting dry and helps connect your internal energy.

So now, you are in a comfortable position and breathing in your nose and out your mouth on a count of four. Continue breathing at this slow steady pace, in the nose and out the mouth. Continue doing this until you are very comfortable with the breathing process. Do this exercise for at least five minutes.

Now, we are going to add something to this. As you exhale, you are to take a certain part of the body and let it totally relax, as if you shut off the switch going to that part of the body. It goes something like this: As you breathe in, think of the tension in the top of your head and as you exhale, turn that switch off and say, "Now, the top of my head is totally relaxed."As you inhale, think of your face and the tension in your face and as you exhale, say, "Now my face is totally relaxed." Now go to the neck and as you inhale through the nose, you think of the tension in your neck and as you exhale through your mouth, relax your neck totally. Turn off the switch going to the neck and say, "Now my neck is totally relaxed."

You continue this exercise and go to the chest, the right arm, the left arm, the stomach, the hips, the thighs, the lower legs, and the feet. You continue turning off the switch to a different part of the body each time you exhale. You do this until you can say to yourself, "Now my body is relaxed from the top of my head to my toes." It is important once you have relaxed a certain part of your body, you leave it relaxed and do not go back and turn the switch back on. This should take about ten minutes once you have learned the technique.

Notice I said ten minutes to learn this technique, not master it. Here is my suggestion: Work only on this breathing/relaxation process for at least two days. You should learn thirty minutes of paradise, or any other part of tai chi for that matter, the same way you would eat a loaf of bread. You would take it in one thin slice at a time and do not work on the next slice until the first slice has been totally consumed. So, for the next couple of days, you should work on using your breath to relax your body. Do not exceed twenty minutes a day, and at the end of the twenty minutes, please do not just jump right up and start running around. Get up slowly and come back to reality slowly.

By now, you should feel comfortable with the physical relaxation part, now for the mental part. We are going to add the mental part in the mix as a part of the plan, not as a separate entity all its own. This is where tai chi differs from other types of meditation which centers on the mind only and separates the mind from the body. In tai chi, the mind and body are always as one.....always.

So, here it goes: You are in your comfortable position. Breathing in your nose and out your mouth and your body is very relaxed. At this point of relaxation, you will stop thinking of anything, especially anything that causes you stress. As you breathe in, think of a stressful situation you are in and as you breathe out, visualize that situation leaving. Do not let it come back in your mind during this time. As you go about dismissing all negative thoughts as you exhale, you next dismiss all thought. You think of nothing. If a thought enters the mind, dismiss it immediately with the next exhalation. This will take some work. Many of us have busy minds with many things going on in our lives. If you keep trying, you will succeed. As with relaxing the body and its muscles, take a few days to work on emptying the mind of all stress using this breathing technique. To be honest, it will take some time and practice. But, if you stick with it and practice about twenty minutes a day, you should be getting the hang of it within less than a week.

Now, you combine the skill you have acquired of relaxing your body from head to toe and mix in with it a total relaxed and empty mind. Notice, please, that you mix it together. You do not add one on top of the other. In other words, the body is relaxing and the mind is clearing itself all at the same time.

It may take a few weeks to a couple of months to get good at this. Start off slowly, with the breathing, then add physical relaxation, then add mental relaxation and dismiss all thought and then do it all at the same time.

You have seen this technique in actual practice if you have ever seen a true martial artist, regardless of their style or discipline. When approached by an attacker, a martial artist will immediately go into a completely relaxed mode. There is no tension, no thought, no emotion…all this at once literally in the blink of an eye. This is the very state of mind and body you can reach that gives you the thirty minutes of paradise.

Only two more things to add to this exercise and the plan to attain thirty minutes of paradise will be complete.

The next step I call creating your bubble. This is how it works: Pick your favorite color. Mine is red. Now picture yourself standing or sitting and you are completely surrounded by that red bubble. Nothing can get in that bubble. Bad thoughts, noise, yelling kids, annoying people, disease, heat, cold, nothing else can get in that bubble and get to you. You can see out the bubble, but no one can see in. So no matter how silly or sad you look, no one sees it.

Now, inside your bubble, do your breathing exercise resulting in total relaxation.

Next, we will add movement to it. If you have been sitting or lying down, now is the time to get up because here comes our first movement, our first tai chi move.

Stand up as if you are waiting in line at a fast food establishment or waiting for a bus. This, I call a natural stance, the "waiting for the bus" stance. Look at your feet and place them just a little more than shoulder width. Stand erect, just like a soldier at attention. Now take this posture and bend your knees slightly, take the part of the body you sit on, your butt, and tilt it forward so it is tucked underneath your spine. Your head is still erect, just like the soldier at attention and your shoulders are relaxed. There is only one more thing. Now you must take your arms which are by your side and bend them slightly as if you were trying to make a letter "c" with your arms. At this point, your hands are at belt level and since your arms are slightly bent, your hands should be at your belt buckle. For some better understanding, go to chapter 11 and look at illustrations 1 through 4. To recap: Feet are a little more than shoulder width, legs slightly bent at the knees, back is totally straight from the tip of the spine to the base of the head and shoulders are down and relaxed and your arms are slightly bent. In tai chi this is called the opening posture sometimes known as wu chi.

From this posture, you form your bubble in your mind and begin the breathing exercise that was just explained. You find something to stare at such as a spot on the wall, a spot on the floor, the red light on you cable TV box, anything that will not move. Remain in that posture and do not move until you are mentally and physically relaxed, and I mean totally relaxed and at peace with the world. This wu chi posture is more than a posture, it is an attitude. During this posture, you forgive everyone and dismiss all worries that may range from a parking ticket to a serious family problem. You stand there until every muscle and tendon and nerve is relaxed from head to toe. You will hear sounds you did not hear before; some even hear their heart beating. During this time you simply stand still and make no moves and listen to your body. In a little while your body will tell you it is time to start moving.

The first move is called beginning tai chi. You look at the finger tips on your hands, push your hands away from your body and then slowly raise both hands together up as high to the top of the shoulder and then lower your hands back down to the point where they were at the beginning of the posture.

Do you remember in the posture that your knees were bent? They stay bent until you raise your arms and as you raise your arms; your knees straighten out slightly, allowing the body to rise with your hands. When you start to lower your hands down to the hip area, your knees bend again and your body sinks with the sinking of the hands.

Breath control is of utmost importance here. You breathe in the nose as your hands and body rise and you breathe out through the mouth as your hands and body sink downward. Each time you lower your hands and breathe out, you try to relax a little more.

Here is the way to properly practice this: You stand in your wu chi posture until you are completely relaxed and at peace, while breathing properly in the nose and out the mouth. By now, you should be wrapped in your private bubble. From your wu chi posture you start moving both hands upward and stop at shoulder height and then lower hands to waist level. As you raise the arms, you breathe in and lift the body and as you lower your hands you breathe out and let your body sink by bending the knees.

This exercise, once learned properly will take about thirty minutes. Did I say thirty minutes? Yes, there is your thirty minutes of paradise.

From doing this one exercise, you are exercising all major muscles in the body: feet, legs, stomach, arms, back, neck and shoulder. You are exercising them, not beating them up as in step aerobics or running a marathon. The proper breathing in sync with the body moves will increase your blood circulation and give you more energy. The relaxation techniques that are coupled with the proper breathing will lower your blood pressure and give you an overall sense of well being.

By learning this one exercise, you will benefit physically, mentally, emotionally and spiritually. And all of a sudden you realize all this is happening to you all at once. There are few things better in life than to receive all these benefits all at one time. Followers of tai chi have been doing this for centuries.

I have had students who learned this beginning move and that was all they ever learned, but at least they know that. Would you like to go a little deeper into tai chi? That would be nice, because we are going to learn in the next chapter about the Taoist influence in tai chi.

5

TAOIST INFLUENCE IN TAI CHI

It has amazed me through the years, how many different ways people use to describe tai chi. It has been described as moving meditation, yoga that glides, a slow folk dance, self-healing, intelligent exercise, a mystical art form, a Chinese ballet, and on and on it goes.

So, how should you describe tai chi? It is an ancient Chinese martial art with Taoist influence. That is all it is. Many think it is more than that. In modern days, with so much more accumulated knowledge in the field of physics, metaphysics, bio-mechanics and a host of so many other studies in so many institutes of higher learning that deal with the human body, its health, its diseases and its primary movements, some have taken tai chi to an all new level and have broken down every aspect of tai chi into scientific jargon. This is a fascinating study, especially for the highly educated and I find it quite astonishing that these scientists do not study any other martial art like they have tai chi. Just for an experiment, you can investigate the Mayo Clinic and find out for yourself how much time and effort they have invested in the study of tai chi as compared to the amount of studies spent on other types of martial arts and exercise programs, and you will see what I mean. It is always good to learn the scientific explanations. It increases your knowledge and deepens your appreciation of tai chi. It is also a good thing that scientists are finding more and more benefits of tai chi.

To gain the most from your tai chi, it is wise to investigate its past and the influence Taoist philosophy has played in making tai chi what it is. Tai chi is not the only thing that has had a Taoist influence in China. To name a few things: medicine, mental health, scientific inventions, gunpowder, pottery, porcelain, balanced meals, healing techniques, sexual advice, longevity, paintings of classic art, the principles of maintaining balance at all time and the art of keeping life simple are all points of interest that have a Taoist background.

There are some who may object to practicing tai chi because it has its roots in an Asian-based religious philosophy, I respect that, since we all would like to please God. It is not and never has been the intention of Taoism or tai chi to turn anyone away from God. If anything, Taoism turns you to God and helps you appreciate nature and the spiritual characteristics of things. Have you ever heard the expression: "A journey of 1000 miles begins with one step"? That is Taoist philosophy.

If you are someone who is very devout in a religion, that is fine and I am proud for you. I would like to put your mind at ease here and tell you that the Taoist influence in tai chi will in no way interfere in your personal worship. This will be repeated again, but I will say now, Taoism is not a religion. It is a philosophy.

You cannot escape the Taoist influence in tai chi. It is evident in its movements and in all the exercise patterns. Some of these exercise patterns are for health, some are fighting skills. They all contain the Taoist attitude. All ancient martial arts, with no exception, had its roots in some form of Asian religious philosophy. Tang Soo Do began with the Buddhists in Korea, Aikido has its roots with the Shinto philosophy in Japan, Karate-do, also from Japan, is from both Buddhists and Shinto. Where do you go to learn real Kung Fu? A Buddhist temple, that's where.

We, who have been raised in a Western civilization, may have some difficulty understanding how holy men could also be such warriors and strong rulers. Simply stated, that is the way the Eastern society evolved throughout the centuries.

I, for one, am quite glad we have the influence of Taoism in tai chi. That is what makes tai chi special and what sets it apart from the act of just standing in the middle of your living room and waving your arms. Taoism is like a ribbon that weaves through the movements and thoughts of tai chi and holds it together as one unit of study. Taoism is to tai chi what a head coach is to football. It is the driving force, the part that gives you the inspiration to carry on even when it is difficult. Without the guidance of Taoism coaching us, tai chi becomes just another exercise we do in order to stay busy after the senior luncheon. All the health and relaxation techniques spring from the Taoist influence in tai chi.

It should come as no surprise that Taoism is all in itself a lifelong study and the purpose of this book is not to be your guide through all the characters and wise sayings located in the Tao Te Ching. We are, however, going to go into some detail of how the wise sayings in the Tao Te Ching have a positive influence on the practice of tai chi, and therefore, can have a great influence on your life as well.

But first, let's study a little about its philosophy and how it may differ from what you may have been taught.

Often, many in Western society will do good things for their fellow man and will be honest and upright in all their dealings because they believe it will have a direct bearing on how they will spend their afterlife. There are others who are assured that they will have a good life in heaven because they have shown a great deal of faith in God throughout their lives. In other words, many of us reading this book have been raised to believe that if we show proper faith in God and are good to our fellow man, it will determine our outcome in the afterlife. You may have even been raised to believe in a heaven and a hell.

Taoist philosophy is different from that approach. It teaches that we should be primarily concerned with our life on earth, because our outcome depends on it. In other words, you will be paid back for the good things you do in this life time while you are still alive on this earth. You will be paid back for the bad things you do as well before you die, not after you die. That is why in tai chi as well as Taoism, we are encouraged to have a strong healthy body, eat right, exercise well, and be calm and respectful toward others. Although there is a path to heaven in the Taoist philosophy, it is not achieved by faith, but rather by hard work, self discipline, respect and many good decisions.

Western philosophy makes a definite division between the spiritual life and the physical life. Taoism does not. There is a balanced blend between the spiritual person and the physical person. The spiritual person is not superior to the physical person, but they blend together even though they are different. This is made manifest by the yin/yang philosophy.

Taoism has no agenda. It has no hierarchy or priesthood as we think of it. Taoism has no gods to please.

It is a way of being spiritual without being sanctimonious.

It is a unique blend of being spiritual while at the same time being physical and scientific. It is a collection of words of wisdom that go back to the dawn of mankind, but was written down by Lao Tzu in the 6th century BCE. It is a balanced philosophy that can add to your happiness and yet it has no savior, no priesthood, and no clergy. That is what Taoism is.

I am sure you realize that there are volumes and volumes of books on the subject of Taoism. I am sure you also realize this is not a book designed to be the ultimate go to book on Taoism. I am including only enough information to help you appreciate the importance of Taoist influence in tai chi.

One other thing before we get started on its influence on tai chi: Like beauty, Taoism is in the eye of the beholder. In Church, it is not uncommon to see two people believe two different things when reading the same scripture. It is called interpretation. No two people describe a mountain the same, explain a scripture the same and, likewise, explain Taoism the same. Because someone else sees it in a different light, that does not make it wrong, it makes it different.

So, let's take a few verses of the Tao Te Ching and see how its philosophy applies to the practice of tai chi.

There are 81 verses in the Tao Te Ching, and if I compared it to anything you may be familiar with it would be the "Book of Proverbs" or, perhaps the "Sermon on the Mount" The Tao Te Ching contains wise sayings that deal with everything from how to pick a flower to how to rule a country. We are going to focus on a few verses that help reveal the secrets that are behind the mind set and personality of a serious tai chi student.

VERSE 8: THE HIGHEST GOOD

"The highest good is like water, nourishing life effortlessly, flowing without prejudice to the lowliest of places."

Tao Te Ching makes many references to water. In this case, it refers to the fact that although water is life giving and beneficial, it often moves to the lowliest of places. Water winds up in the sewer system, in a mud hole, in a dirty marshland or swamp. In other words, even though water is so beneficial to us, it still is not beyond getting "dirty and downright nasty" if necessary. If you were asked to do something that would result in you getting very dirty, such as clean the bathroom at the at local service station, or clean out a septic tank for a friend who had no money, would you do it? No doubt, to perform a task that may be undesirable is always a test on your character and requires much self-discipline. Tai chi is no exception. As a student of tai chi, there will come times when you will be bored, but you still must press on and practice. There will be times that the moves may prove too difficult and you want to quit, but you don't. You continue to practice. There may be times when you feel you are placed in "the lowliest of places", but you press on and you are willing to do whatever is necessary to perform the moves. That is how character is built, by dealing with the "lowliest of places" to the point that regardless how difficult it may seem, how dirty the job appears, we do it. Not only do we do it, we are glad to do it.

Another thought about water being in the lowliest of places is this: When it is in the lowliest of places, it is out of sight, isn't it? You probably travel over a storm drain or a sewer pipe or a manhole cover every day and not once think of the water beneath your feet. It is secret, out of sight, not noticed. Tai chi, from a martial arts standpoint, should be like that. Any martial artist who is an authentic martial artist should be like that. It does not matter if they are tai chi chuan, kung fu, shotokan, tai kwan do, judo or whatever. A true and pure martial artist will never bring attention to himself, but rather would prefer to be un-noticed in a crowd. They are happy to be "in the lowliest of places". This does not mean you should never talk about your tai chi, but it does mean you should never brag about your tai chi, or any other martial art. I have seen young men and women close to my house after tai kwan do class stop at a convenience store for a drink and they walk across the parking lot and in the store and go throughout the store wearing their karate uniform and their black belt tied around their waist. Why are they doing this? Are they showing off their black belt? Do they want to be sure everyone in the store knows they are black belts? Why do these people wear their black belt in public as if it is a piece of jewelry? Are they ignorant of an ancient tradition? No doubt, they have not been taught the proper protocol. Clearly, they know nothing of the principle of staying "in the lowliest of places". They do not realize the importance of keeping a low profile and never appear to be bragging about your rank and your accomplishments. Now, what does that say about their instructors? For a certainty, their instructors did not instill in their students the discipline required to achieve a proper attitude in public. It seems many instructors today either do not know any better themselves or have no regard for ancient tradition.

Bruce Lee said, "You must be like water." If you are a karate or tai kwan do student and you must stop on the way home, at least take off your belt before you get out of the car. If you do this, you will appear to be humble and you will not look so ignorant about ancient ways. This brings up another point. There are no belts in tai chi. Belts limit knowledge. In tai chi, the knowledge is forever, a constant flow, just like water.

VERSE 26: SEDUCTIONS

"Inner strength is the master of all frivolities. Tranquility is the master of all agitated emotions. Those who succumb to frivolities have lost their inner strength. Those who succumb to agitated emotions have lost their tranquility. The wise cultivate inner strength and tranquility. That is why they are not seduced by addictive temptations."

If nothing else, the practice of tai chi will promote inner strength and tranquility. It is called an "internal art" by some, and rightfully so. Tai chi will teach you to focus inwardly to your very soul, to the origin of your energy and emotions. You are taught to strengthen yourself from the inside out. All the while you are focused on the inward self, you are training to be totally relaxed, as you are getting stronger physically and mentally.

It is this inner strength blended with tranquility that has helped some of my students keep their medical condition under control. It is the same principle that has helped other students remain calm in stressful situations.

Now, think about how this can apply to us. Here we are reminded that if we maintain our inner strength and tranquility, and we are approached by negative emotions or by a serious temptation, we will overcome these problems and feel better about ourselves and will come out victorious with a feeling of possessing great integrity. This is how most of us feel after a tai chi class. If we could wave a magic wand and everyone is this country lived their life according to the principles in verse 26, we would not have much of a drug problem, would we?

This tai chi can do for you; provided you have proper instruction and you exert the proper effort.

VERSE 68: THE ETHICS OF WAR

"The best soldier fights without vengeance, without anger and without hate. He puts himself humbly below his comrades, thereby eliciting the highest loyalty from them. This is the power of non-belligerence and cooperation. It is the ancient path to the Great Integrity."

The Taoist philosophy of war is there should be no war. According to Taoism, there is one and only one reason for war, and that is to defend your homeland against attackers. If you **must** go to war, the mindset of the solider should be one who has no emotions toward the enemy. If a soldier defeats one hundred men by the end of the day, it should make him humble, not arrogant.

Tai chi chuan is a martial art and as such, I teach it as a martial art. The philosophy of the martial art portion of tai chi is identical to Taoist philosophy about going to war. As students of tai chi chuan, we never want to fight. We never will provoke a fight. If necessary, we will defend ourselves against an attacker. You cannot hurt anyone with tai chi techniques unless they attempt to hurt you first. It is strictly for self -defense. There are no offensive moves in tai chi like there are in various forms of sport karate that are seen in karate tournaments throughout the world. It contains techniques that will only work when someone is attacking you and, the harder they come, the worse they get hurt. I will give you a quick example of what I am talking about. Have you ever seen a Steven Seagal movie? If not, make arrangements to view one and try to get one made back in the 1980s or 1990s. I give you fair warning: These movies are "R" rated and contain some street language that could offend some. If that is the case, ignore the language and watch the martial arts portions. If you notice, when Mr. Seagal is under attack, he never makes the first move. He always reacts to the assailant's moves. His style is not called tai chi, but it has many of the same techniques and the same philosophy. His style, called Aikido, simply originated on a different island and has a different dialect.

If ever attacked, you empty the mind of all fear and emotion and totally relax the body, as in in "Thirty Minutes of Paradise"(Chapter 3). That will enable you to defend yourself in a most astonishing way. To do this is truly the "ancient path of integrity".

VERSE 78: APPEARANCE AND REALITY

"Nothing in the world is softer and weaker than water. Yet there is nothing better for subduing all that is harder and stronger. Everyone observes how weak overcomes strong, how gentleness overcomes rigidity. How soft overcomes hard. Yet this principle is seldom put into conscious practice."

Verses 76, 77 and 78 all discuss the notion that "soft overcomes hard". If there is one phrase that sums up the very essence of tai chi, it would be these three verses, and in particular, the one phrase "soft overcomes hard". Again, Lao Tzu, refers to water. This time he stresses the fact that water is soft and will give in and take any form. Water is soft, rock is hard. Yet, in time, water will wear down and erode the rock. Calm is soft, chaos is hard. Yet calm will overcome chaos. Have you ever witnessed a large man who is using foul language and smoking a cigarette put out his cigarette and clean up his language when a child enters the room? Soft overcomes hard.

Legend has it that, in ancient China, on the battlefield if there came a time to amputate a soldier's arm or leg, they could have four men hold him down or they could get a young, pretty maiden to sit by his bedside and hold his hand.

The idea that soft overcomes hard permeates tai chi from beginning to end and it is the only martial art that is influenced by these Taoist ideas. It is one of the few throughout the world that uses a soft style; using internal energy as its mainstay. The notion that "soft overcomes hard" has caused many to argue that the soft style of tai chi chuan is superior to the hard style offshoots of karate from Korea and Japan. Today, I am not going to settle that argument. However, I would like to challenge you to settle this argument for yourself.

In tai chi, when you are standing still, you are never rigid. Your arms and legs are always relaxed. Your joints are never locked. There is always a slight bend in the knees, elbows and wrists. When you move, it is always smooth, slow and graceful. When you are practicing your postures, you are always relaxed and calm. You are never pumped up, jumping up and down and yelling and screaming. When you finish a tai chi session, you feel refreshed, energized and somehow just feel better about yourself. That is what soft overcoming hard is about.

From a fighting and self-defense standpoint, the idea of soft overcoming hard permeates these moves as well. In class, the moves are not called self-defense moves. They are call applications of the postures. When practicing, the person you are practicing with is not called the attacker, he/she is called your partner. If your partner throws a punch at you, you do not try to block it with your arm. That would be force meeting force. In tai chi, rather than meet force with force, you re-direct the punch and guide the attacker in another direction, such as to a parked car, a tree, into a wall or on the ground. And here is the good part. The bigger and faster the attacker is, the harder they are going to hit the tree, car, wall, or the ground.

When I boxed, there was an expression, "The fight is won in the mind before the first punch is thrown." I firmly believe this. Your attitude and thought patterns mean everything. From a self-defense point of view, here is where tai chi really shines. Tai chi contains the attitude of soft and yielding will conquer all that is hard and resistant. It contains the mental and physical relaxation techniques that are second to none.

In ancient days, each village was constantly under threat of being attacked by a neighboring village. This made even pulling weeds out of your garden something you did with some apprehension. In today's world, it is unlikely you will be physically attacked while weeding your garden, but a few self-defense moves are still nice to know. And, we still live in a dangerous world. I view the self-defense applications of tai chi the same way I view my car insurance. I hope I never have to use it. But if I do, I am glad it is there. And if you are going to take the time to learn self- defense, learn tai chi chuan. It contains self-defense methods that will serve you well if you are young or old, slim or heavy. It can serve you well throughout your entire life. Maybe that is why they call it the "the supreme ultimate". You think?

VERSE 76: LET YIN PREDOMINATE OVER YANG

"When we are born, we are soft and supple. But when we perish, there is no more tenderness to be cherished. When plants are young, they are pliant and fragile. When they die, as they lose their green, they wither and dry. An inflexible army seals its own fate. When a tree branch grows brittle, it easily snaps."

Again, we are reminded that soft and yielding equals young and healthy. I think back to 1972, when I watched on TV those elderly Chinese men who had the moves of someone half their age. It was the tai chi practice that was the cause of their youthful appearance. The opposite of soft and supple is hard and brittle. As we age, things begin to "stiffen up" a bit. And now, time has marched forward and I find myself close to the age of those elderly men that I watched on TV back in 1972. And now, I find myself doing movements of people half my age. I am so thankful to have had tai chi throughout my life because it has made such a difference in how I feel and what I can do on a daily basis.

Aside from proper rest and nutrition, tai chi is the best when it comes to reversing the aging process and the very best at keeping you young as long as possible. That is because in every tai chi move you are stretching parts of the body and when you get to the end of the form, you have stretched all your muscles, literally from head to toe. Each time you stretch, you open up the molecules in the muscles and allow more oxygen and nutrients to enter the muscles. You are not only making your muscles more flexible, but you are making them stay healthy longer. This is one of the main reasons tai chi is so good for your health. It keeps you "soft and supple".

I have told my students, "If you avoid red meat, eat plenty of vegetables in the correct order, get proper rest and practice your tai chi every day...... you will grow old and die like everyone else. However, you will look a lot better doing it and will enjoy your life much more."

I hope that by reading this chapter, you have a better understanding of the Taoist influence that makes tai chi special and sets it apart from all other martial arts. I encourage you to learn more about the Chinese philosophy that makes tai chi "above it all".

And as far as embracing Taoism goes, do not worry about it interfering with any of your religious beliefs. I once had a very prominent religious leader in Atlanta as a tai chi student. He was a graduate of Emory Theological Seminary and has one of the largest followings I have ever seen. His church has a seating capacity of 5,000. On the subject of tai chi and Taoism, he said, "If it was so bad and so displeasing to God, he would not have allowed it to thrive and flourish for thousands of years." Enough said.

In addition to the Taoist influence, we have a few other things that make tai chi special. Learning these skills are just as important as learning the moves. The next chapter will discuss how to cultivate our chi, perfect our breathing, maintain balance at all times, the yin yang and more information about the good by-products of tai chi.

6

THE CHI IN TAI CHI

WHAT IS CHI?

Chi, pronounced chee, is many different things to many different people. Chi is often misunderstood, not often explained properly. Then, add into the mix that many Westerners have not been exposed to a detailed, accurate explanation of chi, and often the result will be confused opinions and, sometimes a debate based on little accurate knowledge.

The purpose of this book is to acquaint beginners with the basics of tai chi and to instill in all a deeper appreciation of tai chi. That having been said, we are mainly going to discuss how chi is involved in the practice of tai chi. You will find in time that you can only go so far in tai chi and advance no farther until you learn how to develop your chi.

It doesn't help much that there is not a word in the English language that defines chi. It has been referred to as: a force, intrinsic energy, invisible field, aura, soul and even some have told me it was just trickery. It doesn't help much either that many Americans or others in the western hemisphere do not believe chi even exists. These people range from the very educated doctors and surgeons to the very uneducated and narrow-minded. On the other hand, try to keep this in mind: While Europe was enduring the Black Plague and constant attacks from barbarians, Chinese doctors were curing major diseases by strengthening the body's chi. While we were coming up with names such as Plymouth Rock and Jamestown, the Chinese knew how to control pain, even childbirth pain, with the proper guidance of chi through acupuncture.

I have learned from experience that chi is in the eye of the beholder. It has no absolute, carved in stone definition. It is just there. It is there for you to tap in to, it is there for you to cultivate, it is there for you to observe, it is there for you to heal.

Another thing I have learned from experience is this: If you truly want to learn about chi and what it can do for you, you must think like the Chinese and embrace their philosophy and quit thinking like an American. So far, there seems to be no room in the America culture for the total belief in chi.

Thousands of years ago, Taoists formulated the idea that there is an invisible force that moves throughout the universe. This power is the supreme ultimate. There is nothing else like it in the universe. This power is constantly on the move and never rests and, although it is invisible, it can be seen in everything all around you. When you enter the Yin/Yang into this formula, you now have two forces and not just one. These two forces are constantly moving through everything and resulting in a positive force and a negative force. For example, you can have a soft wind that will move a boat, generate electricity, dry your clothes (yin), or a hard wind like a hurricane that can destroy (yang). These two forces are constantly working together in balance and harmony but at the same time are in opposition to each other. It is the yin and yang force that is responsible for the origin of everything in the universe. It was this yin/yang force that began the construction of our planets, our earth, and our sun, everything on the earth and everything else all the way back to the beginning of time. This helps explain why everything is constantly changing. Our world is changing, the universe is changing, and you are changing. You may not be able to tell, but you have changed since yesterday. If you did nothing yesterday, today, you are a little older, a little weaker. If yesterday you practiced tai chi for an hour and went to your first computer science class, you are a little stronger and a little smarter today than you were yesterday. It is this constant movement between the two forces of yin and yang that causes all the changes we see. Nothing stays the same. Your house, your car, your relationships, your appearance, your home town, your planet and all that is in it is a little different today than yesterday. You are in a state of constant change, everyday. Some days you change for the better, some days for the worse. But, nevertheless, there is always a change. That is what chi does, it changes and moves around.

Since this yin/ yang force, called chi, is in the entire universe and it flows through everything in nature, it flows through us as well. That is because we are a part of nature. We are a part of the scheme of things in the universe and as such, we have this chi force moving through us. The only difference between the chi that is in us and the chi that is in an eggplant is we have a brain that can control and direct the chi. Here is where tai chi enters the picture.

To understand chi and how it works and how to cultivate it and even to learn to be aware of it is very important in your journey through the world of tai chi. As you might suspect, you can only advance so far in tai chi without this chi force and then it becomes just another organized exercise program. To study tai chi and learn the moves and not get acquainted with the chi within you makes about as much sense as buying a car without a battery and never putting a battery in it. There is no power, there is no life force, the car is all but useless without the battery; and likewise, tai chi is all but useless without chi.

Would you like to do a quick and easy demonstration on how you can discover the chi in your body? All righty then, here goes: Sit in a quiet place where you know you will not be disturbed for the next ten minutes. Throw your cell phone in the back yard. You don't have to throw it in the backyard, but do turn it off and take it off your body and place it somewhere else. Now take about five minutes to relax, breathe a slow rhythm and just let everything go. Once you are relaxed, place your hands together by clapping together twice and on the second clap, leave them together and close your eyes. Now, here comes the fun part. Continue to breathe in a slow, relaxed rhythm and begin to rub your hands together briskly. It is VERY IMPORTANT that at this time you think of nothing but your hands. Do not think of anything else but your hands. If you think of something else, anything else, this demonstration will not work. So, once again, while rubbing your hands together briskly, all thought is on your hands with your eyes closed. Continue to do this for about one minute, but no more than a minute and a half. Now, stop rubbing your hands together and hold them together as they were right after you clapped. Even though you have stopped rubbing your hands together, continue to think about nothing but your hands. Now pull your hands apart about four inches. You will feel heat and tingling between your hands. At this time, while still thinking about your hands, pull them apart until you no longer feel that tingle. Now, push them back together again and stop when you feel the tingle again. Now, open your eyes and see how far apart your hands are. How far apart they are is directly proportional to how much chi you have in your body. Now, since your eyes are open, look around the room, start thinking of something else, look up at the ceiling, and look down at the floor, ask yourself what is on TV tonight and try to answer the question. Go back and notice your hands. The heat and tingling is gone isn't it? Where did it go? Is it trickery? Well, I have met a few who would say, "Oh yeah, that's just some kind of a trick." A tai chi master will tell you the chi went back to the tan t'ien (pronounced don den) when you quit thinking about it.......better answer. The tan t'ien is where chi originates in the body. You could say it is chi's headquarters.

The heat and/or tingling you felt between your hands was chi that your mind directed to that spot. The slow breathing caused you to relax and focus on the chi. The rubbing together created movement which is necessary for the cultivation of chi. It all came together right there in-between your hands.

We have just learned the most important techniques and principles we must master in order to discover our chi and to increase the amount of chi we posses. These techniques can be summed up the following way:

1. Understand the mind directs the chi, therefore concentration is paramount.

2. It is of utmost importance to relax the mind and body.

3. It is imperative to learn how to breathe properly.

4. You must have your mind, body, and breath in sync as one unit.

5. Next, learn to put all of the above together in your tai chi movements.

6. Simple, isn't it?

THE MIND DIRECTS THE CHI, THEREFORE, YOU MUST CONCENTRATE

The mind is an amazing thing, the most amazing thing on this earth. We all learn when we are young that our minds can make us sick. Certainly sick enough to stay home from school. And then, around 3:00 p.m. all of a sudden a miracle occurs! There has been a cure for this illness! The patient is now well enough to go outside and play. In other words, we already know that the mind can make us sick, and it can make us well.

Today, we have gone past our childhood, but that principle still lingers with us. If we allow it to happen, any of us can focus our minds on how bad we feel, the mistakes we made, the money we don't have, the energy that has left us, and we can spend all day feeling bad. When I met my wife, she was in her 20's. She was thin, tan, athletic and full of fun and humor. She loved to watch football on TV, especially professional football. She was born and raised in Atlanta, and just loved the Atlanta Falcons. She would watch the Falcons game every Sunday and fully expected them to win. (mau ha ha ha ha !) More often than not, they would lose and frequently in the final three minutes. After such a loss, I have seen her quite literally get sick and have to go to bed. One day I said, "You know, football is not worth getting sick over. For the most part it is a bunch of guys who are way too big to do anything else and if they couldn't catch a ball and run fast, they would be lucky to get a job at the post office. There are so many other things we can do on a Sunday that would make you happy and not sick". So, we had five children. Then, her attention drifted from football to the joy of raising a family. Instead of getting sick on Sunday, she was in the back yard running and playing football with the kids. Thirty years have passed since she would become ill over a football game. She still does not get sick because of a football game. Her mind is directed somewhere else.

The mind directs every movement we make, every emotion we feel.

This principle is quite true when applied to tai chi in general and to the development of chi in particular.

As stated earlier, the mind directs the chi and concentration is paramount. So here is a simple exercise for the mind which will improve concentration: Sit in a comfortable position. Find an object that does not move that you can continue to look at. This may surprise you, but I use a yellow crayon. Many use a lit candle. The Goat Keeper (chapter 1) used the red light on his VCR. You sit and gaze at this object for a few minutes until you have this object firmly fixed in your mind. Let's just continue with the yellow crayon lesson. You must now look at the clock and then sit with your eyes closed and in the dark quiet of your mind you see only the yellow crayon. This is the only vision in your head. You continue with this vision in your head and this vision only. Time will pass and eventually you will think of something else. When you do think of something else, do not get upset, it is only natural. When you think of something else, open your eyes and look back at the clock. How many minutes went by? Two? Three? Ten ? Well however many minutes went by is how much concentration you have. Most can last about two minutes at first. Now that you have opened your eyes, look back at the yellow crayon until you have its image firmly planted in your mind, then look at the clock and close your eyes again and try to keep the crayon image in your mind longer. Keep doing this practice until you can think of the yellow crayon exclusively for at least five minutes. Do not exceed ten minutes. If your mind can remain focused on the yellow crayon for five minutes, then your concentration skills are good enough to start cultivating chi.

The next exercise is also for the mind. It is called visualization. In any tai chi move, unless the mind first visualizes the move, you can never make the move correctly. Visualization is the key to success in making the right tai chi moves and is the key to success to cultivating and increasing your chi force.

Back to the quiet, dark room. Sit and be calm for a minute and just breathe normally and slowly. Your hands can be folded in your lap, shoulders relaxed. Now close your eyes and breathe in your nose slowly and out your mouth slowly. For most people, this would be on a rhythm of a count of four. You may feel more at ease with a faster or slower pace with your breathing. Right now, the key is to select a breathing rhythm that is most calming and the least effort for you.

Once your rhythm is established, close your eyes and as you breathe in, pretend the air you breathe in represents a red fog. It does not have to be red. It can be your favorite color. Mine happens to be red. So for sake of discussion, let's go with red.

As you breathe in this red fog, you visualize it entering the body and this red fog flows slowly straight down to an area right below your navel, between your navel and your pelvic area. This is called the tan t'ien. It is the seat of chi in the body. It is where the chi force begins. Again, like the battery of a car. In your car, the energy starts with the battery and then goes throughout the car: to the lights, the wipers, the starter, the music system and so forth. All these items are controlled by various switches. The chi in the body is quite similar. It starts in the tan tien and travels throughout the body and you control it with your mind and send it along its way by turning on various "switches" in the body.

When I was a child, I would amuse myself by dropping a rock in a pool of water and watch the ripples go out in all directions at once. This is how we often teach the way chi moves through the body. The imaginary rock is dropped in the tan tien and ripples of energy race throughout the body in all directions all at once.

So that, in one hundred words or less, is an explanation of the tan t'ien. If you are spending less energy than you are taking in you gain weight, right? Where do you gain weight first? In the stomach and pelvic area. Where is the tan t'ien, the seat of energy? Well, duh, it is in the same area. How about that. Now back to our red fog.

While this red fog is in the tan tien, it swirls around this area and as you breathe out through your mouth, you visualize this red fog leaving your body and it is a little darker than when it entered. This may seem awkward at first, but in time it will be easy and natural. The main technique to keep in mind during this exercise is to keep your breath in sync with the visualization of the red fog. In other words, when your lungs are full, the red fog is deep in the tan tien. When your lungs are empty, the last little bit of fog just left the body. This is called harmony.

This breathing/visualization exercise I just mentioned would be good to practice for about a week to ten days and then we take the next step. The next step is to bring the red fog in as you breathe in and let it circle through the tan t'ien and then while you are still breathing in, send this red fog up from the tan t'ien and through both arms and to your finger tips. In time you will feel a tingle in your finger tips. That is the mind directing the chi force.

To take this one small step further, it is the power of the mind directing the chi force to various parts of the body that causes healing to take place. When you have mastered directing the chi throughout the body, you can now concentrate on one specific part of the body for healing. As an example, let's say you have a bad knee. As you breathe in, you direct the chi, in the form of the red fog, to the tan t'ien and then to your bad knee. Visualize the chi force swirling around the knee and doing what is necessary to fix the problem. Then when you exhale, the red fog is a little darker. This symbolizes it has cleaned out impurities in the knee. Throughout the years I have witnessed this healing power of the chi force many times. It really works on everything from cancer to an upset stomach. The healing power of chi that accompanies tai chi is there for you to use. It is up to you how hard you are willing to work at it. It may not heal the world, but I have seen it heal quite a few.

Also, keep in mind it is a team effort. Relaxation, proper breathing, directing the chi force with the mind through concentration, and then putting all this together with tai chi movements is what will result in healing the body.

As mentioned earlier, concentration skills are quite necessary here. As you visualize this red fog entering and leaving the body, you think of nothing else. You cannot direct this fog through the body and be thinking of your car payment or about how smart your grandchildren are. You have replaced the yellow crayon with red fog. And just like the yellow crayon, if you think of something else, begin again.

RELAX THE MIND AND BODY

Total relaxation is required to get in touch with your chi force and that goes double for doing anything with the chi once you have discovered it. Once you have mastered relaxation, you can not only feel the chi force within you, but you can direct it anywhere. You can direct it to any organ in the body, to any muscle in the body, to any medical problem in the body. You can even direct your chi force outside your body into something or someone else. Before any of this "chi directing" happens, you must first learn total relaxation.

Have you ever been sitting on the sofa, totally relaxed, about to fall asleep and the phone rings and it jolts you. You almost "jump out of your skin"? Has that ever happened to you? I am using this shared experience to prove a point. That point is: the more relaxed you are, the more awareness you have. On the other hand, have you ever been tense, perhaps in a heated argument with someone and the phone rang and you didn't even hear it? So, we learn the more tense we are, the less awareness we have.

Remember I said tai chi is a martial art with Taoist influence and that is all it is? How can it be a fighting skill, a martial art and be so relaxing? How does it happen that many people study tai chi in modern times just for relaxation and stress relief? That is because relaxation is a by-product of the ancient art of t'ai jing ch'uan.

General Chen did not sit one day and tell Yang: "You know, I am so concerned that the mayor of our village is so uptight and the peasants have been throwing temper tantrums because of the high prices in the market. Wouldn't it be nice if we just stopped everything we are doing and taught them to relax?"

Not quite the way it happened. Chen and Yang both knew the more relaxed a fighter is the better fighter he is. A relaxed fighter has more awareness about his surroundings, which could save his life. A relaxed fighter is quicker and smarter and survives better. Have you ever watched a boxing match and the two boxers come to the center of the ring with their trainers to shake hands and come out fighting? Did you ever notice all the while the boxers are receiving their final instructions in the center of the ring, they are rolling their necks around and their trainers are massaging their shoulders? Why? The trainers are trying to keep them relaxed because the more relaxed they are, the faster their hands.

So, we are going to use tai chi principles that you would learn in a real tai chi class and we are going to take these principles and apply them to total relaxation.

As we discussed in chapter 4, "Thirty Minutes of Paradise", relaxation is a mental, physical and spiritual process that happens all at once. And just so you will know, it takes some time practicing these tai chi methods before you can be adept at total relaxation. In fact, if all you learn during the first year of tai chi is how to relax, you can be proud of yourself and know you have done quite well. Tai chi is not a quick and easy fix and neither is relaxation. It takes time to master. Well, I guess we better get started. Time's a wastin'.

Back to your dark quiet room; and I hope it has a nice bed or comfortable sofa or at the very least a clean floor, because we are going to be lying down on our back at the beginning. As far as lying on your back goes, many say it is best to lie on the floor because it stretches the spine better. I do not totally agree with this because for some the actual act of getting down on the floor and getting back up again will negate all the relaxation you just accomplished. Experiment around and learn what is best for you and stay with that.

So, you are in your dark quiet room and you have arranged to have no interruptions for the next thirty minutes, correct? Correct. Now you engage in a process I call turning off all the breakers. In your home or office you have an electrical panel and if you open the door to that panel you will see a row of breakers that are placed in the panel, usually two rows running parallel. They often look like big black switches. These breakers can be turned off just like a light switch. A breaker will control a specific circuit, such as a bedroom circuit, or any other portions of the house. If you want everything in the bedroom turned off, you turn off the breaker that controls that particular circuit. Who is in control of this breaker that just made the bedroom dark? You are.

This relaxation technique has much the same principle in play.

For sake of discussion, we are going to lie quietly in the center of the bed (or on the floor, if you like hard stuff and enjoy getting up and down and being uncomfortable). As a position, you should be on your back with your feet spread apart a little more than shoulder's width, feet in a comfortable position. Place your hands by your side with the palms up. Your jaw should be relaxed with the mouth opened slightly, but not opened to the point where your lips are apart. Your head is tilted slightly forward, thereby pulling the neck straight. Breathe slowly, through the nose only, and do not pay any attention to your breathing, just breathe naturally.

After getting in the correct position, you start "turning off the breakers". By that, I mean you take every muscle individually in the body from head to toe and turn it off, as if you were trying to make this muscle as soft as possible. Allow your mind to direct this shut down and take no shortcuts. There are lots of muscles in the foot, in the leg, in the hand, and so forth. You are in charge. You control the complete relaxation of all these muscles. Some who have studied Chinese healing strongly feel the relaxation should start at the feet and work your way to the top of your head because so many important nerves and channels of energy end in the feet. Let me help solve this dilemma. If you are going to turn off of the breakers in your house, does it really matter if you start turning them off at the top of the panel or the bottom? Not really. Some may argue it would be best to start at the top of the panel, but the results are the same. The power is turned off. The same is true with these relaxation techniques. The point is to relax. In the meantime, we can let all the experts argue which way is better. I like going from head to toe. The other way might work better for you. The important thing is to relax.

Once you have achieved this totally relaxed state, what should you be thinking about? Well, let's think about the ex-husband and how mean he was, or the ex-wife and how expensive she is. Or better yet, how about thinking about the bills! That would be just super, wouldn't it? Not exactly. You should think of nothing stressful. Think of a peaceful situation. My favorite is the sound of the ocean. Use this time also to turn inward. Listen for your heart beat, your breath. Use this time to feel the chi. That is how you relax the mind once the body is relaxed.

This relaxation technique is somewhat different from the "Thirty Minutes of Paradise" mentioned earlier. The thirty minutes of paradise can be done standing up and even while moving your arms and is not a total shutdown. This is more of a total relaxation where everything is completely shut down. Some yoga instructors and some tai chi instructors as well refer to this as "the corpse". That seems to be a good name for it because you are about as still and unmoving as you will ever be until you are a corpse. Once you have achieved this state of total relaxation you will hear sounds not heard before you started the process: a clock ticking in the other room, the fan motor in the air conditioner has a squeak, leaves rustling in the trees from the breath of a gentle breeze. At this stage of relaxation you are more aware of things around you on the outside and you will be aware of your chi on the inside. It is during this stage of relaxation that the realization on chi begins.

There are two other points you should know about this relaxation technique. 1. In this state of total relaxation, your body will do more healing during this exercise than it will do the entire rest of the day put together. That is nice to know if you are sick or injured. 2. Once you have achieved this state of relaxation, you must not just jump up and start running. You come out of it gradually, take it easy. It took a while to get that relaxed; it will take a while to come back to the real world.

Someone completely new at tai chi, named Grasshopper, once asked, "Do we have to do the corpse technique each time we want to get in touch with our chi?" "No, you do not, Grasshopper", says old master Phil. "You see, my little flower bud, the more you do any exercise, the better you become at it. So the more often you relax, the better you can be aware of the chi force. The practice of tai chi alone will help you to relax. The corpse technique will give you more assistance in discovering your chi and becoming a healthier person."

So far, we have learned a little about the definition of chi and that the mind directs the chi with the utmost of concentration, and you must have a relaxed mind and body to discover chi and to cultivate chi.

Next to consider in reference to building our chi force is proper breathing techniques.

IT IS IMPERATIVE TO
BREATHE PROPERLY

Have you ever thought it a bit odd that we pay a lot of attention to what we drink? We pay more than the usual attention to what we eat and how we eat it, and yet hardly any of us pays any attention to how we breathe? What I find even more ironic is: of the three, eating, drinking and breathing, which of these can we live without the longest? Well, it is obvious. We can live for a month or longer without food. We can live for a week without anything to drink. However none of us can live but a few minutes without breathing. So, I ask you, which is more important, to learn how to eat and drink properly or how to breathe properly? Clearly, all are important. But it would be more important to breathe properly.

An easy way to observe proper breathing is to observe your cat or dog. When a cat or dog is lying on the floor and breathing, what is moving, the chest or its stomach? You can easily see it is the stomach. Why is that since the lungs are in the chest? That is because these animals naturally breathe properly using a method called diaphragmatic breathing.

Most people use their chest muscles to expand their chest and thereby take in air in the top part of the chest. This is called the "opening the rib cage and filling the smallest part of your lungs with air and no wonder you are tired and sick a lot of the time", method of breathing. Some refer to it as shallow breathing. This shallow breathing is not good for you because not only are you restricting your supply of life-giving oxygen, but you are maintaining the majority of your lung capacity with stale air that never gets out. Just for fun, let's add a dash of cigarette smoke, a pinch of pollution and two cups of laziness and we have made a recipe for an unhealthy life.

I know of some tai chi instructors who will not let you enter the regular tai chi class until you have completed a course in the proper way to breathe. Some even have Chi Kung (also spelled qigong) classes for the expressed purpose of teaching you how to breathe. Although I do not operate my school in that fashion, I can agree with them and I see their point in emphasizing the importance of breathing.

By Chinese standards, breathing is an art and an acquired skill and a privilege to learn. That being the case, in my schools you earn the right to master the art of breathing after you have begun learning the form. Once you have shown me you have the discipline and the determination to learn, which is reflected in how well you learn the form, and then you are taught the art and skill of breathing.

Let's get started on developing our breathing skills.

As with so many other things in this book, an entire chapter, if not an entire book can be devoted to the art and science of breathing. In fact, I have conducted an entire seminar before just on the art of breathing. There is breathing for power and strength, breathing for energy, for healing, for relaxation. There is even specific breathing for sexual skills and childbirth. We are just going to focus on a small part of it that will apply to your tai chi practice.

Visualize in your mind for a moment a clear, empty glass and you are going to pour in this glass grape juice. How does the glass fill up? It fills from the bottom up, doesn't it? The air in your lungs should fill the same way; namely, from the bottom of the lungs to the top.

You can sit, recline or lie down to practice this: You breathe in and allow your diaphragm to sink. You will notice your belly is pushed outward. This will allow air to enter the bottom of the lungs first. Then you continue by opening the chest and rib cage and allow the air to enter the middle of the lungs. Then you raise your clavicle and bend your shoulders forward slightly to allow air to enter in the very top of the lungs.

To breathe out, reverse the process. Thinking back to the glass, when you empty it, the grape juice leaves from the top first. So, when you exhale, you release the air in the very top first, then the middle and then release the air in the bottom by pushing up on the diaphragm. Thoroughly push up and push all the air out. This removes all the stale air from your lungs. You may feel somewhat dizzy at times, but not to worry; that is poison and impurities leaving the body.

Many teach, when you practice your breathing, you inhale through the nose and exhale through the mouth with the lips only slightly open. Also, place the tip of the tongue to the roof of the mouth. This action helps connect the chi and helps prevent a dry mouth. This is good advice, but not totally necessary when doing this practice. Your are mainly focused on learning (or should I say re-learning) how to use your diaphragm.

Just for the record, it is not a good idea for pregnant women to practice this diaphragmatic breathing.

Other than pregnant women (Why do they always say pregnant women? Are there any pregnant men out there? And if there were, wouldn't the same apply to them?) As I was saying, other than pregnant women, this is an excellent and healthy exercise. It massages your internal organs and gives them renewed life. It all but doubles your air capacity. It slows down your breathing, slows down your heartbeat and lowers blood pressure as well.

And here is the funny part. We were all born breathing this way. When you get a chance, watch a baby breathe when it is asleep. You will see what I mean. As we grow older, we get lazy and get out of the habit of breathing from the diaphragm and just breathe in a very shallow manner.

Another quick and easy exercise is to do an exercise called 'the monkey hang". Stand up, place your feet a little more than shoulder width and hinge at the waist and slowly let your head drop while your hands hang in front of you. Now take in a deep breath through the nose. While bending over and breathing in deeply, you will feel the diaphragm sink. Exhale through the mouth and you will feel it rise.

After you practice your diaphragmatic breathing for a while sitting or lying down, you will feel comfortable with this and be able to do it standing up or squatting or while doing your tai chi moves.

This type of breathing should be practiced not only in tai chi or in your quiet room, but as a way of breathing all the time. According to many tai chi masters, you will live a longer, healthier life if you constantly practice the art and skill of breathing. I totally agree.

So far, we have learned to direct the mind and concentrate while we visualize the chi force in our body. We have learned to relax so we can be more aware of our chi, and we have learned how to breathe properly, which will help chi flow more easily. Now, one last thing: put it all together.

PUT YOUR MIND, BODY AND BREATH IN SYNC AS ONE

This is much easier than it sounds. Think of making a daiquiri. You place the ice, daiquiri mix and alcohol in a blender. You have three distinct things until you turn on the blender and all of a sudden those three things become one.

The mind, body and breath become as one when your mind tells you to do a certain move, such as step forward and your breath is in time with the move. Here is how: you take in a breath from the diaphragm, then step forward and as you are stepping forward, you exhale. That's it? Yes, that's it. I told you it was simple.

This simple principle of harmony coupled with relaxation is what cultivates your chi energy. The final step of cultivating chi force in our body is to put all this together in our tai chi move. That is why it is called tai **CHI** because the postures and moves promote chi.

PUT IT ALL TOGETHER WITH TAI CHI MOVES

Quite honestly, you will find it all but impossible to learn to perfection tai chi moves from a book or a DVD, for that matter. You need experienced guidance. That is because a DVD, or any kind of video production, is two-dimensional and tai chi is three-dimensional. There is always the back side you are not seeing. The same holds true for a book if you look at the pictures and try to follow along. However, I believe you are way above average intelligence and I am going to take you through a tai chi move and you can use this move to develop your chi power. Follow my words.

Stand naturally with your back straight and your head erect, like a soldier at attention. Hold that straight posture with both hands at your side, very relaxed arms. Now, step forward with the left leg in a stance that is natural for you. Lean forward, shifting your weight forward on your left leg, back straight. At the same time move your left hand from your waist and raise it in front of your face, palm toward you, as if looking in a pretend mirror. Take your right hand and move it beside your waist, belt height, with the palm down as if you are petting a dog on the head. This is called parting horse's mane. While parting horse's mane, you exhale as you step forward, empty the mind and gaze at your fingertips on the left hand. Now then, you step back to your beginning natural stance and inhale as you do so. Then repeat the process, exhaling as you step forward and inhaling as you step back. Each time you step forward, relax a little more and do not think of anything but your moves and continue to gaze at the fingertips on your left hand. Now switch sides. Do the same thing only the right hand leads this time.

I can promise you if you do this tai chi move just as I stated, and you incorporated your breathing, relaxation and concentrated on your finger tips, in about 15 minutes you will feel a tingle at your finger tips and your hands will be warm, if not hot.

You have just cultivated the chi force in you and directed it to your hands using the power of the mind, the skill of relaxation , the art of breathing, all coupled with the movement of tai chi. I encourage you to use it well.

If you followed the suggestions in this chapter to the letter, you will be stronger, healthier and happier. You will have something you can carry with you every day for the rest of your life.

SIMPLE, ISN'T IT?

What I mean by that statement is you should not make this complicated. Since most of this may be new to you, it may seem complicated, but it really isn't. You can take one small step at a time until you are able to put it all together.

One final word about cultivating your chi: You never try to make it happen…… relax and let it happen.

This concludes Chapter 6. In these six chapters, I have done my best to share with you certain points about tai chi that I think are important for you to know. Which is the most important point? I can never answer that. That would be just like asking me which is my favorite child. I can't choose one. This having been said, the next chapter is my favorite chapter and, if I had to choose, I would say this is the most important point about tai chi. The next chapter discusses balance. Enjoy.

7

MAINTAIN BALANCE
AT ALL TIMES

What tai chi has done for me more than anything else is helped me to maintain balance. Balance and the role tai chi plays in maintaining balance is important enough for it to be the title and over-all theme of this book.

There are three different avenues of balance:

1. Bio-mechanical balance
2. Physical balance
3. Mental/spiritual balance

BIO-MECHANICAL BALANCE

Bio-mechanical balance is what you have when you don't fall down. As we age, this type of balance becomes more and more important. I remember a TV commercial that ran for quite a while where an elderly lady had lost her balance and had fallen to the floor yelling, "Help, I've fallen and I can't get up!" This commercial ran for quite a while and was very popular. It seems there were some comedians who made this experience a source of humor, as well.

However, falling is no laughing matter. According to the Center(s) for Disease Control in Atlanta, GA, falling is the leading cause of injury and death in one third of the people over 65.

There are several factors that contribute to this: inner ear problems, a decline in muscle strength, loss of eye sight, poor sense of balance and slower reactions all make you lose your balance and make you more prone to fall as you age. Add to this a fear of falling, and a walk to the mail box can turn into a terrifying experience.

For sure, no one wants to live like this, and many do not have to with the help of tai chi.

The keys to fall prevention are to strengthen the muscles, improve coordination and concentration and work on balance training. Clinical studies at Emory School of Medicine in Atlanta, GA, University of Connecticut, Oregon Research Institute and University of Sydney(Sydney Australia) have all proven that tai chi, when practiced regularly, will improve balance by more than 50%. At Emory, tai chi even out performed a computerized balance machine.

A tai chi miracle! No, as in other cases, improved balance is another benefit you receive from the martial art side of tai chi. General Chen was not sitting on his front porch when he noticed elderly people falling down on the path to the village and decided to give them a free seminar on how to improve their balance. Strong postures were built in the tai chi moves to help warriors maintain their balance on the battle field. If we press fast forward from Chen's and Yang's time to today, we realize that we have very little fear of being attacked in our front yard, but we may have a significant fear of falling in our front yard and tai chi is there to help improve our balance.

It is a well established fact that tai chi will help improve your balance. There are no special exercises to do. There is no expensive equipment to purchase. You do not have to see a physical therapist. To coin a phrase, you "just do it". You just do your tai chi on a regular basis and your balance will improve.

According to research in bio-mechanics, it is the heel to toe motion coupled with the constant rocking back and forth that promotes better balance. This simple motion does more for you than you might think. It strengthens your legs and your tan tien area. This is referred to as the "core" in some modern exercise programs. The Chinese were doing core training in tai chi long before there was a United States of America.

In addition to strengthening the legs and tan tien area by rocking back and forth in a heel toe motion, this motion is improving your level of concentration and your blood circulation. As you can clearly understand, if your concentration and blood circulation improves, so will your balance.

When you perform a tai chi move, you are always lifting one foot off the ground and slowly placing it somewhere else, from heel to toe. That means that for a brief second you are standing on one foot. This, too, improves your balance.

I have a balance drill that is quite simple and is exclusive of tai chi, but it works. This exercise goes back to my younger days when I did kick boxing and I was a black belt in tang soo so. You set a timer or look at a clock on the wall that has a sweep hand. Get focused on something, like a yellow crayon.

All you do is lift one leg and no matter what do not put that leg down for 15 seconds.

You see, it is like this: When you were born, your brain told the body that you needed both legs for balance, but you really do not. That is why when you lift the leg in this exercise, you do not put it down until time expires. Even if you have to hop all over the house and out in to the neighbor's yard, you do not put the foot down. If you put the foot down, the brain wins and says, "I told you that you needed both feet, what are you thinking?" No, no, no. You can re-train the brain and make it believe all it needs is one leg for balance.

For people who want to be really good at tai chi, I recommend you do this balance drill until you can stand on one leg for 20 to 30 seconds. This may be more difficult than you would imagine and if you never reach the goal of 30 seconds, be proud of what you can do. You have still improved your body, and that is all that matters.

Another important point to keep in mind as to maintaining balance in tai chi is to be what I call "being centered". Some call it being "rooted" or "well grounded". What this means is your feet should be placed properly on the ground for any posture or move. Tai chi is a martial art, and all martial arts begin from the ground up, standing on a firm foundation. If your feet are not right, nothing else will be right. Even ground fighting styles, such as judo, start standing up with a solid foot foundation. In any martial art, tai chi included, how well you stand, how you place your feet and how well you follow up with good posture is paramount in importance when it comes to balance and relaxation. If the width of your stance is not correct and your foot placement is too far apart or too narrow, you can never be balanced or centered or relaxed. Would you like to know what your proper width would be? Jump off something and land flat-footed on the ground. It does not have to be a very high jump. It can be as high as the bottom step of your porch, no more than six inches or so. You can even jump straight up in the air with both feet leaving the ground at the same time and let your feet land at the same time. Again, I repeat, you do not have to jump high. When you land, look at your feet. That is your proper width. Anything wider than the width you have right now will be a strain on your body and anything that is narrower would result in poor balance.

Keep your knees bent slightly and your feet flat, in touch with the ground. When standing in the wu chi posture, visualize your feet growing roots into the ground. All this, too, will help you maintain balance. It will help you become centered and rooted.

On a personal note, at the writing of this book, I am 62 years old. I can stand on top of a ladder with no trouble. I hike in the woods and on nature trails on a regular basis and never fall. I simply do not have any fear of falling. I owe this good balance to my tai chi.

PHYSICAL BALANCE

Tai chi will give you physical balance as well. Physical balance differs from bio-mechanical balance in that it has nothing to do with falling down. It has to do with both sides of the body being balanced or equal. This means by practicing tai chi, your left side and your right side are equal in size, strength and abilities.

There are some people who are very right-handed and can do nothing with their left hand. To take this farther, this will enlarge to the point where one entire side of the body is weaker and less skillful than the other side. Since mankind, in general, is quite lazy, as people get older, they have a tendency to take the path of least resistance and favor their strong side. In this way, by the time people are in their forties they have become very "lopsided". You may even notice someone sitting in a comfortable position and they are leaning to one side. Look at someone in their forties, say at a dinner party, standing and talking to a friend. If you look more closely, you will no doubt see they are favoring one leg while they are standing up. They either have their strong leg slightly to the rear, or their hips are tilted to one side and the majority of their weight is resting on their strong leg. You will notice this in women more than men because as a group men tend to be more athletic and more physical than women and also, men often wear flat, more comfortable shoes.

This principle even spills over into professional sports. You will see a quarterback who seldom rolls to the left to throw a pass, a professional boxer who has more trouble fighting a left-handed opponent, a soccer player who has trouble playing the right side of the field.

Let me ask you a question. You do not have to be scientist or a medical doctor to answer this question correctly. All you have to be is wise. The question is: "Do you really think that being physically unbalanced is healthy?" If you answered "NO" you have more on the ball than most scientists and doctors in this western hemisphere who choose to ignore the importance of maintaining a physical balance within your body.

Proper balance throughout the body is of utmost importance by tai chi standards. Proper physical balance not only keeps the muscles stronger, but promotes more energy and even affects the health of the internal organs.

Once again, if you practice tai chi on a regular basis, you shall acquire total physical balance. And once again, it is not a tai chi miracle based on some ancient spiritual trip to enlightenment and back. You may be tired of hearing it, but it is a martial art and as such, ancient martial artists were trained to be as effective left-handed as right-handed.

Even today, when I teach my students the self defense side of tai chi, I ensure they become equally skillful on both sides. What if you were attacked in a parking lot and the first thing that happened was you broke your right arm? Are you now rendered useless or do you have plenty more weapons?

Speaking of Yang style tai chi, the underlying theme is balance. You have Yang 24 moves, 48 moves and 108 moves. As you notice, these are all even numbers and that is no accident. It was carefully thought out a few years ago. To achieve total physical balance, it is required you complete the entire form. If you begin learning and quit half through and never go back to class, you will never achieve the balance I am talking about here. As you begin your tai chi moves, you will notice you are always shifting sides. If you do "parting horse's mane" and lead with the left hand, you will immediately turn and lead with the right. Each move is designed for you to work both sides of the body and both sides of the brain at the same time. Even though while you are favoring one side while doing a move, you immediately switch and do the other side. The end result is this: When you have completed the last move in your form, you have equally exercised all muscles on both sides of the body. You have also equally affected all the organs throughout the body.

I have had many students who have had little trouble performing their moves on one side, and find the other side all but impossible. It is normal for everyone to have a strong side and a weak side. We refer to this in tai chi as "a good side and a better side". In time, you will have two "better sides".

For those who have a lot of trouble with one side as opposed to the other side, that is a red flag giving you the message that your physical balance needs improving.

There is only one bit of advice I can give: If you are having trouble on the left side, when you practice you must do the left side three times to each one time you do the right side. In time your body will balance out and you will be as strong on one side as the other.

MENTAL/SPIRITUAL BALANCE

Up until now I have always had a simple explanation for the benefits tai chi offers. Up until now I have always said the benefit can either be traced back to the martial arts or Taoist philosophy. This one I have a hard time explaining. When you finished your tai chi workout for the day, somehow your mind feels more balanced. Your mind is not cluttered with all the mess you had to deal with today. It seems all worries and problems are gone. There is a calm that cannot be described. You just plain feel good all over. This feeling I am describing may happen the first week you begin your journey into tai chi or it may be a year later. But I promise you, that day will come, and when it does, you will know what I mean.

Up until now, everything I have written has been either documented by research papers or by personal experience. What I am about to tell you is nothing more than my opinion. If you have a better idea, tell me and I will enter it in my next book and give you credit for it.

We achieve mental balance in tai chi because we are always working both sides of the body, therefore working both sides of the brain. It is stated the left side of the brain controls the right side of the body; the right side of the brain controls the left. That is why it is said left-handed people are the only ones in their right mind. Ok, I know, thousands of comedians are unemployed and I am trying to be one.

All joking aside, tai chi postures, tai chi moves, and tai chi forms are working both sides of the brain at the same time and this produces a balancing effect within the mind. In addition, as you may recall in previous chapters, we are to empty the mind, totally relax and focus on one thing such as breathing or our fingertips. So now, what we have is a mind that has dismissed all worries and problems and for the first time all day is in a relaxed state and operating both sides in a balanced manner.

It is also my opinion that this is no accident. The Taoists placed this mind balancing benefit in tai chi to achieve not only total physical balance but mental balance as well. In the 16th century, medical science in the western hemisphere separated the mind from the body. Throughout Europe you had physical health and mental health. To the Chinese and others throughout the eastern hemisphere, the mind was never separated from the body in the field of medicine. To this day, Chinese believe it is the mind that heals the body and healing is attained by balancing the chi in the body and not by pouring pills down you.

Tai chi also gives you a sense of spiritual balance as well. Your continued practice of tai chi and the principles of balance that it offers will in time make you feel closer to nature and closer to God himself.

We are a small part of nature; and when we are balanced in mind and body we become closer to nature, which is perfectly balanced. Can you think of an example where for thousands of years a piece of land, such as a great forest, was doing just fine until man came along and upset the balance by dropping all the trees or killing all of a specific animal, such as a wolf? You can read about the terrible dust bowl that plagued this country in the 1920s and early 30s. It was the result of mankind upsetting the balance of nature: killing the buffalo, pulling up all the prairie grass, damming up the creeks and rivers upset the balance to the point we created our own hell.

To properly achieve this spiritual balance, it is best to retreat deep into nature where there is still balance, and practice your postures and your tai chi moves by a waterfall, beside a babbling creek or under a 100-year-old tree. You can even do this in the quiet of day in your own yard.

Keep practicing your tai chi under the direction of a competent instructor that you like, and I promise that you will achieve a balance in your life you never even suspected existed.

No self respecting tai chi author would ever write a book without mentioning the yin/yang symbol. Now is a good time for this, because yin/yang is the universal symbol for balance.

YIN /YANG......THE SYMBOL OF TRUE BALANCE

Every sports team has a logo, every country has a flag and every martial arts style has its symbol, or patch. Tai chi has as its symbol or patch the yin/ yang, and nothing could be more appropriate to symbolize tai chi than the international symbol for balance.

Legend has it that a Taoist sage contrived the idea of yin yang when he saw two fish in the bottom of a round basket and one fish had its head on the other's tail and all of a sudden the yin/ yang came to him in a flash and so did all the philosophy that accompanies the yin/yang. It seems somebody had a good imagination, either the one who created the legend or the sage who saw the two fish.

If you are not the least bit familiar with tai chi or the Chinese culture, you still are probably somewhat familiar with the yin/yang symbol. It is on t-shirts, on billboards, TV ads. I even know a lady who has a yin yang tattoo and she has no idea what it stands for. As you can see in the illustration, the yin yang looks like a perfect circle with the letter "S" drawn through the center. On one side of the "S" is a white figure with a black dot in the center of the larger end, and on the other side is a black symbol with a white dot in the center of the larger end. Come to think of it, it does look a little like two fish in a basket, doesn't it?

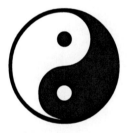

As you can see, there are no corners, no sharp edges, or no angles. It is all smooth curves. For such a symbol to be so simple and have such a deep meaning is nothing short of amazing if not miraculous. But that should not surprise us, should it? Tai chi itself is nothing short of amazing if not miraculous.

Simply stated, the yin yang symbol means all things are balanced...all things. They are balanced by having two opposite forces in them. Let's just give you a few hundred examples. There is good and evil. You would not appreciate the good if there were not evil. The fact that the white half of the symbol has a black dot in it and the black half has a white dot means that there are no absolutes. For example, there is some good in the worst of men and some bad in the best of men. Daytime is appreciated more because it is offset by nighttime. For every hill, there is a valley. You have masculine and feminine, and even though they are opposites, they complement one another and balance each other. You don't really appreciate young until you get old.

Everything in nature, everything in your body and everything in tai chi balances out by opposites. In nature, if we did not have rain, the whole world would be a desert. We have day and night so man and animal alike can have time to rest and time to do its duties of the day. We have beautiful oceans complimented by dry land. What would it be like if we had no oceans? What would it be like if there were no dry land?

In our everyday life, we can enjoy a much healthier and happier existence if we apply the yin/yang to all we do. Have you ever known a "clean freak"? It is far easier to live with someone who is good about cleaning, but doesn't mind a little mess. It is wise to be serious, but maintain a sense of humor. If you are funny all the time and never have a serious moment you are a train wreck waiting to happen. You should not be too fat, or too thin. You should not be too demanding, or be too complacent. To maintain a happy life, you should be neither too rich nor too poor. For those who believe you can't be too thin or too rich, I invite you to study the life of Howard Hughes. He weighed 90 pounds when he died and he died alone and miserable even though at his death, he was worth billions of dollars. Do you think maybe this one-time handsome billionaire could have used a little more balance in his life?

It seems the ancient Taoists were trying to tell us that any extreme is bad for us. We can go overboard with anything: with fitness, with discipline, with wealth, with eating, with not eating. My goodness, you can even drink too much water and drown your own self!

So, let's just maintain balance at all times. Learn when to yield and when to stand firm. If you become the recipient of strong words, fighting words about where you squeeze the toothpaste, ask yourself: "Is this really worth getting upset over, is this worth a serious fight?" Or instead, is it not a better time to balance these strong words with soft, yielding words such as: "You are so right, I guess I was in hurry and not thinking about the toothpaste." Sometimes in a marriage, the yin/yang comes into play, and you just have to ask yourself: "Do I want to be right or happy?" "Is this the hill I am willing to die on?" Also, remember balance is required when it is time to fight instead of time to yield. The Taoist sage who influenced the self-defense side of tai chi designed it so it would work only if you were attacked. Force is only possible when attacked. As a martial art, Yang tai chi is not aggressive, but is very deadly to a violent attacker. Not aggressive, but deadly. That sounds like more yin/yang, doesn't it?

For a certainty, we would not stand still and allow someone to take our child or to try to kill us. That would be an example of being unbalanced in the other direction. This would be too much yin and not enough yang. Other than the aforementioned extreme cases, a calm respectful attitude will conquer more than a belligerent attitude will ever accomplish.

YIN YANG IN TAI CHI

As tai chi students, we learn what the yin yang symbol means. Yin represents the softer things in life, the feminine side of things and is represented by the white side of yin/

yang. Yang, on the other hand, represents the hard side of life, the masculine side of things, and is represented by the black side of yin/ yang. Even the ten major organs of the body are matched up into five yin/yangs. The solid ones are matched up with the hollow ones. The kidney goes with the bladder, the heart with the small intestine and so it goes. Everything balances. It is test time. In music, which would be yin, a sweet lullaby you sing to get a baby to sleep or a high-powered rock and roll song?

Here is another test. Tai chi is a soft style martial art that emphasizes soft overcomes hard. Is that correct? Yes, correct. Now comes the test question. How do you think the yin yang symbol should appear if it is to represent tai chi? The correct answer is the yin yang symbol should appear with the white over the black to properly symbolize tai chi. The tai chi philosophy stands for soft over hard. That would mean yin over yang. Yin is represented by the white half, and therefore white should be over black if it is to represent tai chi in a correct manner.

One reason you need to know this is when you are looking for a tai chi school and you observe their yin/yang symbol is upside down, that is your chance to smile a little and remember the words you just read.

The tai chi student's goal should be to become the line in the center of the yin/yang symbol. We should be completely balanced in the classroom and outside the classroom. The tai chi moves reflect that philosophy.

When we do beginning tai chi in the Yang style, first our arms move upward, then downward; we inhale, we exhale. Can you say opposite moves, boys and girls? Can you say yin/yang? Next is even a better example of total balance. As you step forward to do part horse's mane, your right hand which is on top goes to the bottom and your left hand which was on the bottom, rises to the top. Again we have opposites creating balance and harmony. As you begin to execute part horse's mane, you step forward and place the majority of your weight on the front leg. What comes next? You roll backward and place the weight on the rear leg. Here we go again. We roll forward, so we can roll back. We shift our weight to the front leg so we can shift our weight to the rear leg.

This is another one of those unexplained mysteries of tai chi. The more you practice your tai chi, the more balanced you become. And I mean better balanced in everything. You can stand up better and seldom if ever will fall. Your body appearance and your strength will be equal on both sides. Here is the punch line: You will find in life that on a daily basis you will be a better husband, a better wife, a better student, a better grandparent. You will be slow to anger and quick to help. You will be hard-working but know to relax. You will be kinder and more respectful to your fellow man but less tolerant of wrong doing.

Would you like to have a little more stable life? Would you like to be able to maintain balance in an unbalanced world? If you would, I encourage you to embrace tai chi and its philosophy. Within the world of tai chi is every type of balance that you need.

8

QIGONG, TAI CHI'S OLDER COUSIN

Qigong, pronounced "chee kung" is an ancient Chinese exercise program that is often confused with tai chi. Since it is confused with tai chi, I am adding a chapter in this book to help dispel this confusion.

Qigong is also spelled chi kung, chi gong, and chi gung. I actually prefer the chi kung spelling because it seems to imitate the sound of the Chinese word the best. It is also the most popular way of spelling it in Great Britain and throughout Europe. However, we will take the "when in Rome" approach and call it Qigong because that is the most popular way to spell it in the U.S.A.

Qigong is two words in Chinese: "chi", meaning internal energy and "gong", meaning work, or working at it. Qigong means doing a work that promotes chi force.

The definition alone indicates it is very similar to tai chi, which also deals with promoting and cultivating chi within the body.

Like so many other projects and designs in ancient Chinese culture, qigong was a closely guarded secret for thousands of years. Add to the secrecy, the fact that there are over 10,000 different styles of qigong and you can imagine it is quite a challenge to discuss qigong in a detailed manner to the point where everyone would agree on the material you present. My intention in this chapter is to share with you the differences and similarities between tai chi and qigong. At the end of the chapter, I am going to introduce you to a book and its author that will discuss in great detail qigong and its benefits. Since this is a book about tai chi, not much detail will be offered about qigong. After thorough investigation, you may even decide to study qigong instead of tai chi.

I teach both tai chi and qigong at my school and I have found from experience that many take tai chi when they really needed qigong, but were not up to par on all the information. However, I have never found a tai chi student who wanted to transfer to a qigong class, even when I recommended it.

Primarily, qigong is much older than tai chi as an organized system. But to say it is the great granddaddy of tai chi would be a mistake. It is more like a distant cousin to tai chi. If I wanted to oversimplify it, I would say that qigong is to tai chi what weight lifting is to football. It is the physical conditioning and energy making portion of tai chi.

Qigong also has its roots in Taoism. Furthermore, qigong has, as its primary concern, healthcare. There is a good reason for this. A few thousand years ago when Taoist philosophy was the dominate influence in China, people would pay doctors to keep them well. If they became sick, they would quit paying their doctors. As a result of this, the Taoists priests devised a program that was designed to keep you from getting sick. This program worked the chi force in your body in such an efficient manner that illness seldom came to your door. When it did come, you were so healthy you did not stay sick for any length of time. Did I just say "worked the chi force"? Isn't that qigong? Quite right. Qigong was originally an exercise designed to keep you well and if you ever did get sick, it would get you well rather quickly.

Although some experts disagree, qigong never had that much to do with martial arts. It was and still is a balanced lifestyle that emphasizes good health and healing. Tai chi, emphasizes good health, healing and martial arts. In qigong, a master who is qualified can give you hands on treatment by means of massage and applying pressure to various points in the body and in so doing can perform healing. When a tai chi master places his hands on you, you are probably going to be thrown to the ground.

Many say there are three divisions of qigong: Meditative, Medical and Martial. I do not doubt the meditative and medical part, but in 46 years in the martial arts, I have never once seen someone step forward and say they are an expert martial artist and their style is qigong. I have had qigong people tell me the martial side of qigong did not really mean fighting, but meant making you stronger internally so you could become a better fighter. This makes more sense to me. In the United States, qigong is known for health and exercise, not self-defense.

One thing that tai chi and qigong do have in common is the slow, harmonious moves. Some even look similar if not identical to each other. The main difference in these moves is if you trace the move back to tai chi, it has martial art applications that kept you healthy. If you traced the same move back in qigong, it would have health and healing applications. As I mentioned when discussing the Sun style of tai chi, it is not uncommon for someone to take ideas and techniques from another style and apply it to their own system and create their own style. As to the slow harmonious moves you see in tai chi, were they always slow? No, they were not. Were they changed and made slow to benefit more people? Yes, they were. Do you think perhaps the founders of the slow moves in tai chi may have gleaned the concept of these moves from qigong? That could very well be.

Let me give you an illustration that should help you see the differences and similarities between tai chi and qigong. Throughout the United States, in all major cities, you can find a fitness center and somewhere down the street, you can find a karate school. Most of us have seen kicks and punches preformed by someone in a martial arts film. In the fitness center, you can witness an aerobics class which is full of men and women in spandex outfits and tennis shoes doing kicks and punches to loud, thumping music. Just down the street is a karate school where there is a young man in a karate uniform, called a gi or do bak, and he is barefooted while he is doing these same kicks and punches as hard and fast as he can into a target or focus pad with no music, but with a lot of yelling.

If you asked the aerobics people why the kicks and punches, they would say, "To raise my heart rate and it burns the calories and gives me a good workout." If you went down the street to the karate school and asked the same question, they would say: "It is a part of karate discipline, the faster and more powerful your punches and kick are, the better fighter you become."

So, perhaps you see a pattern here. In aerobics, physical fitness is emphasized, whereas in karate, discipline and self-defense are emphasized, even though the movements are very similar. In qigong, health, medicine and healing are emphasized, whereas in tai chi health and healing are there also, but it is an art for self-defense as well; and the movements are very similar, in some cases. In all these above mentioned cases we have the same moves executed for different reasons in different environments.

Here is another obscure example that you may find interesting. In the medical school of qigong much time is spent studying "dian-hsueh" or pressure points throughout the body. These are power points or special switches in the nervous system that you press to achieve a healing effect. Upon more study, you will find the healing arts of acupuncture and acupressure are both results of this study of "dian-hsueh". In tai chi, as well as other martial arts, this same internal energy system is studied in order to incapacitate and immobilize an opponent. Immobilize and bring down an opponent using only two fingers? Well it is true, and this is how: There are pressure points throughout the body that are stationed at various intersections in the nervous system. In some circles of the martial arts community, these are called "nerve strikes", although that is not a completely accurate statement. There are nerves you strike, nerves you press and nerves you rub back and forth to get the desired result. In martial arts, the desired result is taking down an opponent. In qigong, the desired result is to promote healing. Although both study the nervous system, it is studied for different results.

Upon studying the same nervous system, qigong healers apply acupuncture; tai chi masters apply dim mak. One heals, one disables. Although it is the same nervous system, the results are quite different.

Tai chi has healing principles built into its practice and philosophy and a good tai chi master knows how to heal and maintain a healthy body and mind. He also knows what to do if he were attacked by three thugs in a parking lot. A qigong master may not.

In conclusion, you might say both qigong and tai chi share

the same goals of maintaining a healthy body and mind, but for different reasons. To a qigong practitioner, a healthy body meant a happy life. To a tai chi practitioner, a healthy body meant he could be a good warrior.

If all you want is a good exercise program, it would not make a lot of difference which one you practiced. You would benefit from either as long as you remain dedicated to the exercise and practiced regularly.

Here is the way we do it at my school: If you are over 65 and have not done anything physical for a long time, I strongly suggest you begin in a qigong class, because the moves are much easier to learn. I recommend at least four classes of qigong before you take the first tai chi class because this gives you a jump start on breathing principles with slow moves. In qigong, the learning curve is easier and the pace is slower and there is less to know to obtain a workout. Quite naturally, then, qigong would be better if you have memory problems or have suffered a minor stroke.

Tai chi, on the other hand, requires a good memory and at least average co-ordination. It has also been my experience that most people enjoy tai chi more. I have had some qigong students transfer to tai chi, but I have never had a tai chi student transfer to qigong, even when I recommended it. I said that earlier, but it bears repeating.

I have a special qigong class that meets once a week, where many in the class have serious health problems. The qigong really works for these people. I see it work every week.

As with tai chi, it is sometimes difficult to find good qigong master. I can give you an example I ran into a while back not far from where I live. You will love this one. This is someone from out of state who advertises being a Certified Qigong Medical Master. This person is 40 years old and here are their credentials: A yang tai chi sifu, a chen tai chi sifu, a Taoist Priest, a college graduate, a certified massage therapist, certified in hot rock therapy, and graduated from a school of Qigong Medicine. OK, let's think this one through:

It takes 10 years to be a yang tai chi sifu.
It takes 10 years to be a chen tai chi sifu.
It takes 10 years to be a Taoist Priest, at a minimum.
It takes 4 years to be a college graduate, at least, if you spent no time partying.
It takes 2 years to be a certified massage therapist, some schools require 4 years.
It takes ? years to be certified in hot rock therapy.
It takes ? years to graduate from a Qigong Medical School . This could be one weekend, or it could take many years. It depends on the quality of the school.

This would total to 36 years of study, not counting the hot rock therapy and the Qigong Medical School. That means this individual started their journey to help humanity at the age of four. What an awesome healer! No time for Barbie dolls and G.I. Joes here. I must perfect my yang tai chi before I am eight years old so I can move to Atlanta and start healing people when I turn 40. We met at the studio, oh I mean "healing center", and as this person was walking around their 600 square foot area, I could not help but notice their do bak (top like a jacket that ties around the waist) yes, as I was saying, the do bak was on backwards. I guess they missed do bak day in qigong class. Oh, by the way, the belt was tied incorrectly, too.

The truly sad part of this is the average person, who is unexposed to the Chinese way, might not know the difference between this pseudo healer/master and someone who is genuine. Feel free to question credentials. A true sifu will appreciate the wisdom behind your desire to find the real thing.

One of the best books on Qigong is called: "A Complete Guide to Chi Gung" The author is Daniel Reid. I find his books informative, very detailed, and easy to read.

Here are the particulars:

A Complete Guide to Chi Gung
Author, Daniel Reid
ISBN#1-57062-337-6
Shambhala Publishing
First published in Great Britain by Simon & Schuster, 1998

The next chapter I believe will interest you, and I am certain it will benefit you. It deals with my reflections as a teacher.

9

A FEW WORDS ABOUT TEACHING

I have often said in a joking way, "I have tried all my life to avoid being rich and famous, and so far, I have succeeded." Wealth and fame have not impressed me as much as being a skillful teacher; which brings me to writing this book. I am not writing it to become rich, but to become helpful. Over the years, many students have requested I write a book that could be an easy to follow guide to tai chi. So here I am. I do not like to sit still. I do not like to be in front of a computer, entering words on a word processing program. I can't spell worth a damn and my wife wants to use the computer. Nevertheless, here I am, sitting in front of the computer day in and day out writing these words as they come into my head. I am doing it for one reason and one reason only. I am doing it for you. I am positive there is something you could read in this book that could help you, and that is why I am writing it……. to be helpful.

That brings up the reason for this chapter where I shall say a few words about teaching. Most of these words have been taken from the instructor's edition of a textbook I wrote a few years ago. I have found these principles apply in a dojo, a tai chi classroom, and most importantly, throughout life. Perhaps you can use some of these words in your teaching, or just getting along in life. These words I say to you are principles, and as such you can carry these principles wherever you go and no matter who you are. These words, I believe, are helpful.

First of all, I believe good teachers are born, they are not made. There are natural born salesman, natural born athletes, and even natural born healers. We all have a gift and a purpose in life and the sooner we discover what that purpose is and pursue that purpose with all our heart, the happier we will be. However, this does not mean you cannot teach, but it does mean you may have to learn how to teach, if teaching does not come natural to you. For example, you can teach an electrician how to be a vacuum cleaner salesman, even though his heart is in electrical work, he can still sell vacuum cleaners. Likewise, you can still teach, regardless of your calling.

So, here are seventeen principles that deal with the art of teaching:

1. Never forget that 2+2=4 was brand new to all of us at one time. Just because it is easy for you, does not mean it is easy for your student. Try to remember this one. Especially if you ever teach your daughter how to drive a five speed manual transmission automobile.

2. Always try to think like a brand new student would think. Often they are excited, unsure, completely ignorant about tai chi or the martial arts, and are unknowing. Sometimes they are very concerned about their physical condition and sometimes they are just plain scared.

Always teach through their eyes, not yours. In life, try to see through the other person's eyes.

3. Never show off your techniques in front of a beginner. You must remain humble. Those who enjoy showing off in front of those either less experienced or less skillful are headed for disaster.

4. As with teaching the martial arts, so with life, the key ingredient is respect. Treat older ones like your parents, younger ones like your children and treat all as if they are better than you.

5. Teach the same way you would feed steak to a small child. You should cut off one thin slice and let the child thoroughly chew it and swallow and then give it another small slice. Teach tai chi or anything else one small slice at a time. Of the two, it is better for a student to leave wanting more than to be overwhelmed with information and become discouraged.

6. Try to remember the five ingredients that make a successful teacher, a successful person: Patience, Understanding, Superior Knowledge, Superior Techniques and Superior Attitude.

7. Be a wise teacher and never criticize a weakness a student may have, but instead realize all are different and all have differing strengths and weaknesses. Dwell on their good points and praise them for that. There is nothing to gain by dwelling on anyone's bad points. This is true in the classroom and throughout life.

8. Never show favoritism; love them all the same.

9. Do not abuse the power and authority you have as a teacher. Remember the example set by Jesus Christ. He was above it all, and yet chose to

be among the most humble of men. So should you.

10. This may sound off the subject, but find hobbies and interests that will expand your mind and teach you something new. I enjoy going to historical sites and museums and spending the day learning something entirely new and different. Where I live, in the Southern United States, there are hundreds of nature trails and state parks that are rich in Civil War History. It just feels good not only to get away, but to learn something new while getting away. Regardless of where you live, you are a one hour drive from something you have never seen before. Explore, take pictures and share this with friends. Somehow, this makes you a better teacher if you continue to learn yourself.

11. Always think before you speak. My grandfather once said: "Even a fish would stay out of trouble if it knew when to keep its mouth shut." This is good advice in life as well as in the classroom. Once you say something bad, it takes a long time for someone to get over it, some never do.

12. Discipline yourself first so your school will be disciplined. Always be on time. Always show respect for the student's time by not going fifteen or twenty minutes over the allotted time. Every day, arrive in a clean, fresh-smelling uniform, with a clean, fresh- smelling body and enter a clean, fresh-smelling school.

13. Maintain a simple life and be content with the smaller, simpler things life has to offer. This will allow you to stay focused on your students and what you will be teaching instead of how you are going to pay for all these things you have

accumulated. Let's think back to Jesus Christ, Mahatma Gandhi, Lao Tsu, Buddha, Pope John Paul II. You never found these great teachers traveling the world in their private yachts or running around screaming and hollering in a stadium full of frantic people while wearing a $5,000.00 suit. In fact, if you study these people, you will find they had little to nothing when they died, but the influence they had on the world of mankind could never be measured. Ask yourself: "Would I rather be the richest man in the cemetery, or the best teacher that ever lived?"

14. You must truly care about your students. There are some who profess that there needs to be an invisible wall between student and teacher. That the teacher is somehow more revered and respected if there is a large gap between student and teacher. This is even seen in some churches where the clergy stand high above everyone else by standing in a pulpit or on a high stage whereas the laity sit and look up and listen. Well, they can have it all. I do not agree. I think it is a mistake to think you should not get close to your students. It is a mistake to think you can mold them into excellent tai chi practitioners and see them for one hour a week and then forget about them. Their desire to learn does not end when they cross the parking lot and get in their car to go home. Neither should your desire to help them. Do not hesitate to get close to your students. If you do, they will see you are human and approachable, and that increases the teaching process and makes it better for both student and teacher. And if they realize

you are not something special and godlike, all the better. That is the way the Tao meant it to be. I have held students in my arms while they cried having just learned they had cancer. I have been asked to attend a funeral where I was the only white man in a funeral home full of Chinese. I have been there as I watched a student fight MS. I have been the only person outside the family invited to a High School Graduation of a student that I took a personal interest in. I have had students fix my house, repair my car and take me out to eat. All this and much more simply because I truly care about my students and develop an interest in them not only as a student, but as a person. And just for the record, you can keep the $5,000.00 suits and the yachts. I will keep the love my students have for me. That is priceless.

15. Never under estimated the far reaching influence you may have on a student. My Kenpo instructor, Sifu Ken McGuire, died way too soon in life. He died not long after he promoted my friend, Jim Fuller, and me to 3rd degree black belt. That was in the early '90's. To this day, words, expressions and techniques that he instilled in me are alive and well and used on a daily basis. That is the only immortality we know truly exists. What you say and do as an instructor can last for generations and can influence people not even born yet. Think about Master Chen and Yang in the 1700s. Their influence is still here and it encompasses the entire world. If you practice your tai chi, some of your thoughts will have been their thoughts. So, never think that what

you do as a teacher is small, because its influence can be great.

16. Do not be overly concerned about your appearance or your position. Again, stay humble. Stay balanced as the way of the Tao sets out. I have often told my students: "I do not teach you tai chi, you teach yourself tai chi. I merely guide you through the process." You can compare this principle to the bridle on a horse. It is very small, you can hardly notice it, and yet it can control this powerful animal and guide it anywhere you want. That is a true teacher, one who is in the background and guides the class. Not the one in a flashy uniform with his chest poked out.

17. The last and most important principle about teaching is, above all else, be a good example inside the classroom and outside in the real world. When you take off your uniform and leave the classroom, you do not take off your honor, respect, concern, honesty and balanced approach. You take these qualities everywhere you go.

So here we have seventeen principles of teaching. Why seventeen? Why not eighteen or twenty? It is because 10 + 7 = 17. Ten (10) is the symbol of earthly completeness, seven (7) is the symbol of spiritual completeness.

As stated earlier, I have spent my entire adult life as a teacher, either in karate or tai chi, sometimes both. You will be hard-pressed to find these seventeen principles anywhere else because they are based on my experience. This ,too, I want to share with you from experience: When I leave the classroom and re-enter the real world, I have noticed that the more I behave like I did in class, namely patient, understanding, kind, etc., the easier things go for me. This may help you, also. I have learned from experience that these tai chi principles can expand beyond the classroom and give you a better life. In fact, let's take a few tai chi principles and apply them to daily living.

10

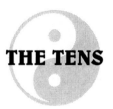

THE TENS

This chapter contains lists of various points associated with tai chi, that, when applied, will give you a better life.

TEN BENEFITS OF TAI CHI

1. It relaxes the muscles while making them strong
2. It removes stress from the mind and body
3. You achieve better balance, mentally and physically
4. You will have better coordination
5. Your posture will improve
6. You will have instilled in you a better feeling of self confidence
7. You will enjoy better flexibility
8. It will improve your concentration, memory
9. You will learn proper breathing, which equals better health
10. It calms the soul and soothes the spirit

TEN WAYS TO ENSURE A
GOOD TAI CHI FORM

1. Practice daily, same place, same time
2. Learn the correct posture and use it in your form and everyday life
3. Keep your muscles loose and soft
4. Do not do straight movements, all movements must be rounded
5. Do not ever lock out any of your joints, keep joints curved slightly
6. Learn to meditate while doing your tai chi form
7. Visualize your moves before doing them
8. Visualize your chi force moving throughout the body as you move
9. Develop good coordination between your feet, hands and breath
10. Develop proper breathing by lowering the chi into the tan tien

TEN WAYS TO ENSURE A
GOOD TAI CHI WORKOUT

1. Try always to go to the same place, same time, with the same clothes
2. Drink a glass of pure water with no chemicals, nothing added such as flavored vitamins
3. Warm the body up with a 10 minute walk, qigong moves, low stance posture, arm movements
4. Loosen all joints, starting with the ankles and end at the neck, loosen all gently
5. Do some basic stretches, especially the lower back, legs and arms

6. Slow relaxing music may help, and is often a plus
7. Continue to slow the body movements down
8. Begin to relax the entire muscle structure from head to toe
9. Achieve the proper mindset: no worries, no outside thoughts, just think of your tai chi moves
10. Begin your first move with a warm, relaxed body and a clear mind

TEN STEPS TO MEDITATION

1. Heard this before? Set aside a certain time and a certain place everyday
2. Give enough time for all the feelings and frustrations inside you
3. Replace those feelings and frustrations with happy, positive things
4. Close your eyes to all that is going on in the outside world
5. Relax by deep breathing, think only of happy, positive thoughts
6. Feel and visualize your breath entering and leaving the body
7. Go through all the thoughts in your mind and make them leave
8. Focus on one thing, let go of every other thought
9. Take time to understand what your mind and body needs, experience the flow of chi in the body
10. Don't use meditation as a quick fix. Anything worthwhile takes time and effort

TEN STEPS TO PROPER BREATHING

1. Breathe in the nose with nostrils slightly flared
2. Breathe out the mouth with lips slightly apart
3. Place the tongue to the roof of the mouth
4. As you breathe in, let the diaphragm sink
5. Let the air rise from the bottom to the top of the lungs
6. As you exhale, let the air release from the top down while pushing up on the diaphragm
7. Always think about your breathing and about how you are breathing
8. Visualize the chi force entering the body as you breathe in
9. Teach your breath to be in time with your moves
10. Remember: You control your breath, your breath controls your emotions and all internal actions

TEN WORDS TO LIVE BY

1. Respect, above all else, there is respect for mankind, the animals, your time, other's time
2. Stand up straight, good posture is everything
3. Never get too upset about things
4. Always be honest with your fellow man, always be honest with your feelings and desires
5. Fear no man
6. Nothing can happen that a calm, confident attitude can't fix
7. Always live in the moment, for the moment. Never try to change the past or worry about the future
8. Treasure everyone around you. God has surrounded you with these people for a reason

9. Stay well grounded, centered, and dependable. Always be a good influence
10. And most important of all, maintain balance at all times

TEN STRETCHES THAT WILL HELP

1. Bend at the waist, let your head hang down and totally relax, rotating arms, then slowly rise up and let your back bend backwards slightly
2. Bend back down with your feet shoulder width, grab both hands to you left ankle, pull your chest to your knees, then go to your right ankle and repeat, 10 seconds each side
3. Spread feet apart about 10 more inches and repeat: grab left ankle and pull chest to knees, then to the right and repeat, 10 seconds each side
4. Take both hands and push them through the center of your feet toward the rear for 10 seconds
5. Stand up, bend your left leg, stretch your right, then reverse, bend your right leg, stretch your left, 10 seconds each side.
6. Squat down with left leg, stretch right with toes up, reverse with right leg, toes up for 10 seconds
7. Hold both arms straight out from the body, like the letter "t" and slowly twist the body to the left and then to the right for 10 seconds
8. Sit in a chair, cross your legs with your left ankle on your right knee, pull up gently on your ankle and make small circles with your ankle, then reverse, do same with the right ankle for 10 seconds

9. Pull your left arm across the body, then right arm for 10 seconds
10. Grab your finger tips and pull back, stretching the wrist, repeat on both sides for 10 seconds

TEN EVERYDAY EXPERIENCES WHEREIN TAI CHI CAN ASSIST

1. If you are in traffic and there is a tense situation, do not allow this tense situation (yang) to overpower you. Instead, remain calm (yin), do your tai chi breathing and relax.
2. If you are in a situation where you will have to wait a long time, such as the airport, at the driver's license bureau, a long line at the drive thru, try thinking about your tai chi moves and put them together in your mind while you are waiting. You will be surprised how quick the time will go by.
3. When a door is stuck and you can't open it, don't just keep jerking your arm, instead, grab the door handle, let the body sink down about three inches and pull back with your entire body instead of just using your arm. You are rocking back just like in the form.
4. If you are having a stressful time at the office, go outside, think of the balance of nature and think about breathing properly. Take time to do this and your day will go better.
5. If you find yourself getting weak and need more strength, such as to climb a hill or a set of high steps, stop for a few seconds and perform deep breathing exercises and you will be happy to notice a new found strength and energy.
6. When you choose a place to live, choose one

that has lots of trees and, if possible, a creek running through the yard. If this is not possible, at least find a dwelling that has a park nearby. This will give you a healthier life that is more peaceful.

7. Some days things just do not go the way we want. Some days are a train wreck. Use the yin yang philosophy in this case and tell yourself: "This bad day can help me to appreciate the good days." And then promise yourself when you go to bed that night that tomorrow will be a good day.

8. When you drop something on the floor, don't fuss about it. Instead, use it as a chance to stretch your muscles as you pick it up.

9. If you play golf or if you are on a softball team or bowling league, there is so much tai chi can do to help. Concentration, coordination, relaxation and making the body move as one unit will improve any of your athletic endeavors.

10. Be careful, don't fall. In everyday life, tai chi will give you the balance that will prevent falls.

TEN WAYS TAI CHI PRINCIPLES CAN HELP A MARRIAGE

1. Be patient. It takes patience to learn tai chi. It takes patience to deal with children and a mate.

2. Stay relaxed. Avoid high stress discussions at mealtime. When high stress discussions are necessary, keep them calm and relaxed. Screaming and pointing fingers accomplishes nothing.

3. Remember, soft overcomes hard...every time.

This one thing could eliminate most of the strife in a marriage. Quiet is better than loud. Slow is better than fast. Kind is better than selfish. To bend is better than to break.

4. Slow everything down. As in the moves of tai chi, so should our life be. Let's see: today I have golf at 9:30, junior has a soccer game at 11:00, and missy has dance at 11:45. The grass needs cutting and we must pay the bills before 5:00 to see if we can afford to go to the movies and out to dinner by 7:00, because we deserve some recreation. See any red flags? See any of yourself?

5. Remain focused. We must keep in our mind a clear vision of the posture and moves when we are doing in tai chi. The same is true in family life. Keep a clear vision of what you want your family to be and do not become distracted from that vision. I once had a student, a devout Christian, and we were talking about home schooling. I made the comment: "You know, home schooling is great, except often the higher educational institutions will not accept home schoolers in spite of their superior SAT scores." He said: "I don't want them to go to Harvard; I want them to go to heaven." A man who is focused is a good man.

6. If you become a serious student of tai chi, someday you will realize that tai chi is a lifelong endeavor. Keep in mind the same is true in raising children. Raising a child is a 40 year project.

7. Allow the self discipline you find in tai chi to spill over into your finances. There are more divorces that are filed as a result of what goes

on in the checkbook than what goes on in the bedroom. Do not be hasty, stay balanced, and keep it simple.

8. Use tai chi principles to avoid fights and heated arguments. I am a black belt in three styles of karate and a master of tai chi. My wife is a black belt in karate, undefeated in competition, and a certified instructor. More than once someone has said to us, "Wow! I bet it is really something to see when y'all get into a fight." My wife or I will always answer, "We never fight." And it is true, we never fight. We maintain a calm respectful attitude toward each other and have for 30 years. We are just like everyone else. We have the problems and pressures that accompany raising a family and operating a business and running a household. We have taxes, insurance, medical problems, death in the family and pregnant daughters like everyone else. We have our share of pressure and stress, but how we handle the stress and problems is what makes the difference. Avoid fighting at any cost, remain calm through it all. Tai chi principles really work.

9. Approach family problems the same way an ancient warrior approached the battlefield: with a clear mind and with no emotion. If you do so, fits of anger, physical beatings, bad language will be in the past. Never be too angry with family members or too complacent. Remember the ancient way and copy its principles.

10. The tenth and most important point in maintaining a happy marriage? You guessed it. Maintain balance at all times. Remember the

yin/yang works as well in a marriage as it does in tai chi.

TEN WAYS TO TRAIN FOR SELF DEFENSE

1. If you are threatened by an angry person, do whatever you can to calm the situation.
2. Remain calm, like water, feel their force coming toward you and re-direct that force.
3. Never meet force with force. The attacker will almost always be larger than you, stronger than you, and will have much anger. But the attacker is never smarter than you. Use this to your advantage.
4. When grabbing an attacker's arm for a takedown, you must go the same speed as the attacker, feel the attacker.
5. Remember, when under attack, the lower your center of gravity the better.
6. If you are under attack, have a calm attitude coupled with no emotion. As long as you are relaxed and can think, you will not panic.
7. Make up your mind now, ahead of time, what you will do and how you will do it. It will be too late to think of this once you are attacked.
8. Keep in mind: "The best defense is common sense" (Jim Fuller's Creed, UMAS Karate). Avoid situations that may place you in danger.
9. If they push, you pull. If they pull, you push. Do what you must to place the attacker off balance.
10. Never give up; "it ain't over until it's over". [sic] Practice daily your self defense applications. Let justice prevail.

So now, I have listed ten different categories in which there are ten different ways tai chi and its underlying principles can help you. Let's see. 10 X 10 = 100. That is one hundred different ways. When I was in school, a 100 was an A. If we follow these principles, we can better our chances of making an "A in life". Maybe even an A+ in some areas. You think?

Until now, all the words in this book were designed with a theme in mind with the overall goal of educating you about tai chi or helping you achieve a better appreciation for the martial arts, or both.

In the next chapter, I am going to divert from my theme and just share with you some neat stuff that is nice to know. The chapter contains a combination of many scattered thoughts that I thought you would enjoy.

11

NEAT STUFF THAT IS
NICE TO KNOW

A GLOSSARY OF TERMS

Balance:
Balance in tai chi is different from everyday balance because it encompasses mental, physical and spiritual balance.

Chi:
The invisible energy inside you and everything else in the universe

Do Bak:
The Korean term for Karate uniform

Dojo:
The Japanese word for classroom, a catch all phrase for any assembly hall

Do Jang:
The Korean word for dojo, classroom or assembly hall

Form:
Also know as a kata, it is a prearranged sequence of moves that are always done in the same order

Gi:
Also spelled ki, is pronounced "gee" is a traditional martial arts uniform

Hard Style:
A style of martial art most notably from Japan and Korea that emphasizes external strength and includes much physical conditioning as well as karate moves. It is characterized by straight ahead kicks and punches that are hard and fast. In self defense, the idea is to meet your attacker with force and overcome with blocks and counter moves.

Horse Stance:
One of the low postures where your feet and legs assume the position of riding a horse with your thighs parallel to the floor

Linage Holder:
Someone who has studied tai chi with a particular family for many years. After many years of study they are considered a part of the family and are given all the techniques and secrets that the family has to offer.

Low Posture:
Any posture that requires a bending of the knee at 90 degrees

Master:
This is a term which holds a great deal of respect in China, but seems to be overused in Western civilization. In China, it is someone who has mastered the martial arts, in this case, tai chi. Traditionally speaking, it takes at least 20 years to master the art of tai chi, or any other martial art. More is

mastered than the martial art. A true master is a healer and a wise advisor as well.

Move:
Any one sequence within a form

Posture:
A position that has a particular shape and form about it, but you remain stationary

Soft Style:
The style of martial art that promotes internal strength instead of external strength. It is characterized by soft, flowing techniques with gentle moves as opposed to the hard and straight ahead punches and kicks of karate. In self defense, the idea is to use the attacker's power and energy against them and divert the attack somewhere else, such as to the ground or a tree.

Sifu:
Pronounced "see foo", the Chinese word for teacher; sometimes also referred to when speaking to a Master, although some refer to a master as Zeefu

Tai chi:
An ancient martial art with Taoist influence

Tan Tein:
Pronounced "don den". The place of origin of the chi force in your body, located below the navel

Tang Soo Do:
A Korean style of Karate that dates back to 700 a.d. Literally translated it means: "Way of the Chinese Fist." Tang Soo Do in its traditional state is known for its circular moving hands and hard, devastating kicks

Taoism:
An ancient religious Chinese philosophy that dates back more than 600 years BCE.

Tao Te Ching:
A holy book of wise sayings written by Lao Tsu which contains the basic Taoist principles

Wu Chi:
The most important posture in tai chi. Wu Chi is used for meditation, relaxation, strength and discipline

Yin Yang:
The universal symbol of balance. The yin yang symbol has its roots in Taoist philosophy which has an overall theme of maintaining balance in all things

TREES IN TAI CHI, QIGONG

It has been observed that trees which bend and sway with the wind are the ones that lasts the longest. Therefore, we can see the importance of proper stretching in our own bodies to avoid getting stiff and non flexible. The tree that hardens and does not yield to the wind is the one that will fall. Likewise, in our personal lives, it is often better to yield and bend rather than be stiff and break. Also, a tree is only as good as the nutrition it takes in. It is likewise with people.

The main reason tai chi/qigong has been practiced for so many years outside is due to the health benefits of performing these exercises in the presence of trees. The old masters teach here is a transfer of energy between man and tree that cannot be matched indoors.

There are several postures in tai chi/qigong that refer to

trees. Hold the tree, hug the tree, sparrow in tree, tree in winter, tree in wind, and be like bamboo , to name a few.

Tree in winter is a posture and a meditative attitude that was designed by master Chen Lam in the 1600's, according to legend. You first assume the posture of hug the tree where your arms are in a circle in front of you and your fingers almost touch, knees slightly bent. Totally relax, breathe properly.

Remember this:"A tree in winter places into the ground all of its life force where all is warm and safe so it can withstand any hardships that winter may bring. You, too, can be like a tree in winter. Place into the ground all your hatred, worries, medical issues, all that causes you stress and strife in your life and if you do this, you, too, will be like a tree in winter and able to withstand anything."

THE NEGATIVE ION ADVANTAGE

A subject that has been researched in the greatest of detail is that of negative ions. In spite of decades of research, few people other than research scientist know anything about them due to a lack of publicity and a lack of educating the general public on the advantage of negative ions.

If you have stood beside a large waterfall or gone outside on a cool clear morning while in the mountains, take in a deep breath and then somehow just feel better, you have received the benefits of negative ions.

What is an ion? Simply stated, it is an atom that has a negative or a positive charge. Normally, the protons, neutrons and electrons provide a balance of charge in an atom, but sometimes things happen to cause an electron to jump from one atom to another which then results in one atom having a negative charge and the atom that lost the electron has a positive charge.

Ok, so much for physics class. Our concern is how negative ions can make you feel better? And make a difference in your life?

We all know what we take into our body effects the way we feel and act. A good cup of coffee will refresh us in the morning and get us going, whereas a glass of wine will relax us and calm us down. How would you like to be refreshed, energized, experience less fatigue and be relaxed all at the same time? Well, that is exactly what negative ions will do for you. When you breathe in oxygen that is rich in negative ions, it will travel through the body and energize your entire system while at the same time have a calming influence on your entire system.

In our breathing practices, the importance of breathing in oxygen rich in negative ions cannot be understated. If you work in an office all day you will be far more physically drained and more stressed out than if you worked in the garden all day. This underlies the importance of negative ions in your life.

Japan and the USA have both spearheaded the research on this subject and have discovered that oxygen beside a large waterfall has 100,000 negative ions per cubic centimeter, whereas an office or crowded expressway at rush hour contains about 500 negative ions per cubic centimeter. This helps to explain why you feel so refreshed outside on a cool clear morning in the mountains and you can hardly stay awake in the office.

With this in mind, many Japanese corporations have installed negative ion machines in their offices and factories and have seen a marked increase in productivity. The USA is doing this also, but not to the extent as the Japanese.

So, the question is: As a serious breather, what can I do to gain the negative ion advantage? Well, you could stand beside a waterfall all day. Now that would be nice. You could spend some time outside each morning for a few minutes doing some deep breathing exercises. That may a little more realistic. If it is impossible to be outside on a regular basis, you can purchase a negative ion machine for your home for about $400.00. You can find them quite easily on the internet.

TAI CHI LINAGE

As mentioned earlier in this book, I promised a graph that would depict the family linage of tai chi. As you study this chart, keep this in mind: Ancient China was full of secrecy, had a difficult language with many dialects, and plenty of legend. You may find this chart a little different from others. In fact, I would be quite surprised to find any two linage charts identical. This is the chart I find to be the most accurate and what I have used to trace my tai chi linage. This graph depicts the combined research of four tai chi masters. To view this graph, see illustration in this chapter.

LEARNING THE MOVEMENTS IN THE FORM

As you may already know, it is all but impossible to learn tai chi from a book or DVD. This is because a book or DVD is two-dimensional, whereas tai chi is three-dimensional. There is always something going on the other side that a book or DVD cannot show. Therefore, a good instructor is absolutely necessary for you to learn tai chi properly.

That having been said, it is my intention to describe to you the opening ceremony and the first move, called parting horses mane. This will give you plenty to work with until you find the right instructor. You will be quite surprised how much there is to learning just that and you will be equally surprised how much benefit you can receive from only learning that much provided you practice on a consistent basis.

OPENING CEREMONY

Opening ceremony is the same as wu chi posture. This sets the stage for the entire form. Wu chi is both a posture and an attitude. As for the posture: Your feet are about shoulder width, knees slightly bent, back is perfectly straight like a soldier standing at attention, the base of your spine, the tailbone is pushed forward underneath the body and the back of the head is pulled upward. The design and intent of this posture is to make the spine as straight as possible. While maintaining this posture your shoulders are curved and relaxed and your arms are curved slightly in front of you with your palms down. Yours eyes are looking down between your two hands, gazing at the floor or ground. To re-cap: back is straight, knees bent, head erect, shoulders relaxed and arms bowed in front of you. That is the posture; now comes the wu chi attitude: as you are breathing slowly, you forgive everybody, you dismiss every worry, all medical problems, all hatreds, all that causes stress in your life... totally dismiss these things from your mind and totally relax.

When you feel inside you have achieved wu chi, namely the posture and attitude, you can move to beginning tai chi.

BEGINNING TAI CHI

Beginning tai chi is the first time you will have moved in the form. With your arms bowed, hands in front of you , palms down, knees still bent, you let your wrists go completely limp and raise your arms up in front of you to the height of your collar bone. At this point, knees should have straightened out by then. Now with your hands in front of you at collar bone height, lower your hands to about four inches below the waist. As you lower your hands, lower the body by bending the knees. That is beginning tai chi. Next comes hold the ball.

HOLD THE BALL

The object of this posture is to give the appearance you are gently holding a beach ball next to your chest/stomach area, while placing all your weight on the right leg. The top hand should be about three inches below your collar bone and the bottom hand should be about three inches above your navel. Here is how you do it: As you lower your arms and body in the beginning move, you keep your knees bent and you begin to separate your hands at waist level…..looks as though you are rubbing a counter top with your palms. Take your left hand, turn palm upward and let it sweep across the body and allow it to stop in the center of your body right above your navel. As you sweep this arm across the body, you also allow your left foot to slide with it and bring it to the top of your right foot. It should give the appearance that there is a string attached at your left wrist to your left ankle and when the hand moves, the foot moves with it. The arch of your left foot should now be resting on the top, or instep, of your right foot, with all our weight resting on the right foot, right knee still bent. At this point, if your right leg is trembling slightly, you are doing it right.

And now for the right hand: The right hand turns its palm

up ward and with your right hand you draw a large circle in a counter clockwise motion and allow it to arrive in the center of your chest right below the collar bone with palm facing down. You now have achieved the posture called holding the ball. As you hold this posture, visualize in your mind a swirl of energy between your hands where the imaginary beach ball is. In time, you will feel heat or a tingling sensation in your hands.

Do not go any farther. Practice this move over and over until you can do it without thinking about it. To be good at this posture, practice it daily for about twenty minutes a day for one week and then you will be ready for the next move called part horse's mane.

PART HORSE'S MANE

From the position of hold the ball, while still standing with your body weight on the right foot only, knee slightly bent, turn your head and look to the right, then look to the left.

As you look to the left, you twist your left shoulder slightly to the left as well and then begin to move the right hand which is on top. You move this hand until your knuckles are even within the end of your shoulder. Pretend you are reaching out with your right hand to grab a tree branch that is shoulder height.

Remember the left foot that has been resting on top of your right foot? Now you move it as you move your right hand. You lift your left foot about ½ inch above the ground and place this foot straight in line with your left shoulder, placing the heel down first.

Now, you begin to shift your weight forward to your left leg. As you do this, take your right hand and pull it down to your side, about waist high. Your palm should be facing down, arm slightly curved. It should look as though you are patting a tall dog on the head with your right hand.

At the very same time, you move your left hand, which was above the navel. You move it upward at a 45 degree angle until it is shoulder height. It should look as though you have an imaginary mirror in your left hand and you are looking at your face in the mirror.

That is Parting Horse's Mane. Well, that is as least the beginning of Parting Horse's Mane. Now we do the other side.

From the position you just finished, shift all your weight back to your right leg and slide your left leg back about three inches and pull the ball of the foot up on the left foot where just the left heel is on the floor. This is called rollback position.

As you roll back, you take your hands and make the holding the ball position on the right side of your body. At this point, your left hand should be on top, making the top half of the ball, and the right hand is about waist height on the bottom half of the ball.

While still holding the imaginary ball in place, you twist your entire body 180 degrees to the left, twisting the feet, hips and shoulders.

At this point, you are facing the other direction, holding the ball this time with the left hand on top. Now you part horse's mane the same way you just did, except now you are on the other side. You reach out with your left hand and pull it down to your side about waist height. In other words, you are patting the dog with the left hand this time. At the same time your step forward with the right foot. The right foot goes forward, stepping in line your shoulder. Step with the heel touching first. As you are stepping forward with the right foot, the right hand rises at a 45 degree angle and ends in front of your face as if it were a mirror. These three steps, when perfected, will happen all at one time. For now, you may want to do just the hand techniques and then add the foot movement once you have learned the hands.

Cheer up, we are almost finished. Now that you have done Part Horses Mane on the left side, we shift and turn and do Part horses Mane on the right side one final time.

Right now, your right hand should be in front as if looking in a mirror, left hand down by your slide, patting the tall dog. Now, it is time for another roll back.

You shift all your weight to your left leg while you pull your right leg back about three inches and bring the ball of the foot up on the right leg.

Now, you bring your hands back to the hold the ball position. It looks just like you are holding a large beach ball on the left side of the body. The right hand is on top about shoulder height, palm down and the left hand is about waist height, palm up.

Once you have shifted your weight to the left leg, and you are in the hold the ball position, you twist feet, hips and shoulders 180 degrees to the right.

Now you are right back where you started. You move the right hand out past the shoulder. Pull it down to the waist. Step forward with the left leg, heel first. Take the left hand which was down beside the waist and bring it up at a 45 degree angle and it should be in front of your face. The imaginary mirror again.

You have just completed Opening Ceremony, Beginning Tai chi and Part Horse's Mane. What you have just learned represents about one month's work in a tai chi school. So do not be surprised if it takes you a minute or two to learn these moves by looking at a book without any outside supervision.

What I have just shown you is a gracious plenty to get you started in your pursuit of learning a tai chi form. There are many who learn this and nothing more and find it to be a great exercise of great benefit.

To help you understand the moves somewhat better, I have provided some illustrations. You can see them on the following pages.

ILLUSTRATIONS

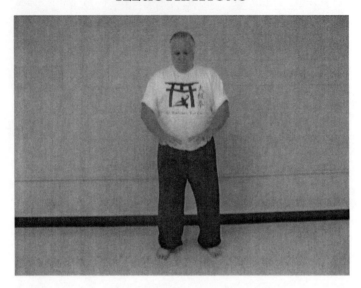

1. Wu chi

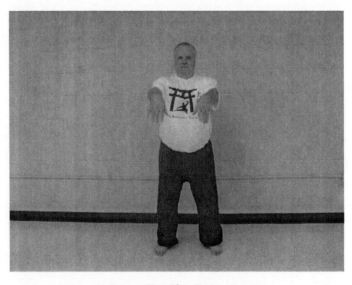

2. Begin Tai Chi, Raise Arms

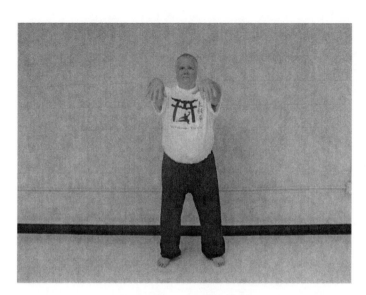

3. Raise Arms to Shoulders

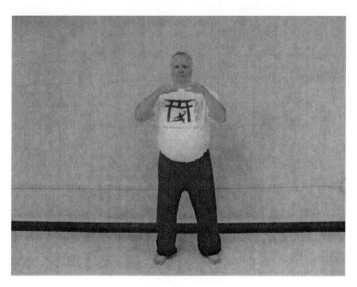

4. Push Down

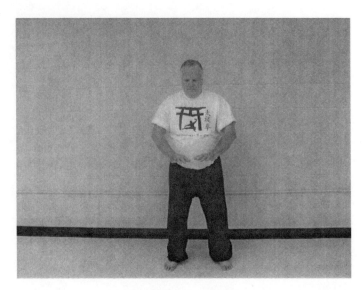

5.Push Down to Waist

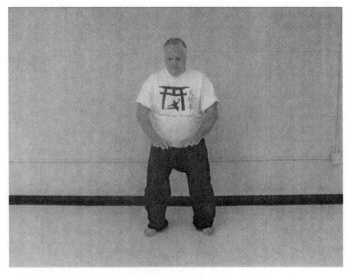

6. Let Body Sink

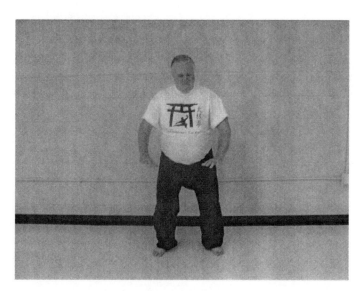

7. Seperate Hands

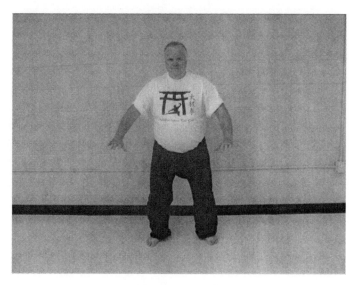

8. Seperate Hands, 2

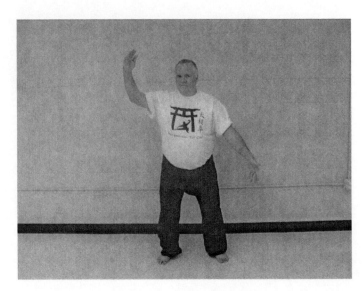

9. Begin to Hold The Ball

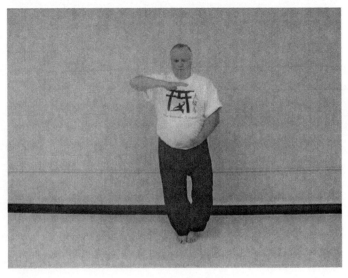

10. Hold The Ball

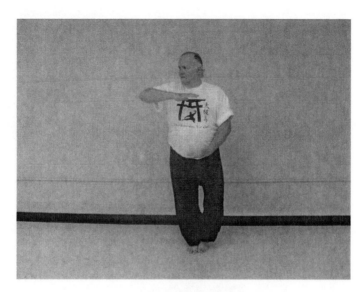

11. Look to the Right

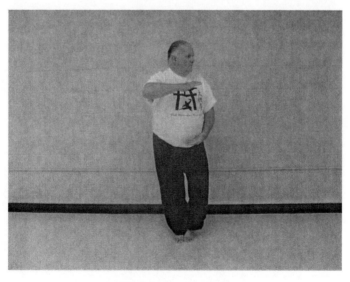

12. Look to the Left

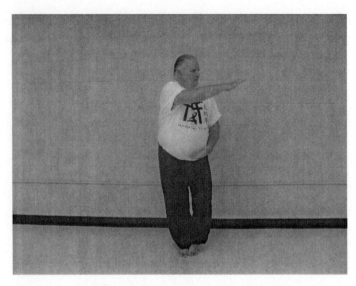

13. Right Hand Moves Past Shoulders

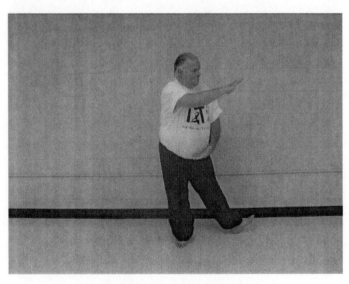

14. Step Foward With Left Leg

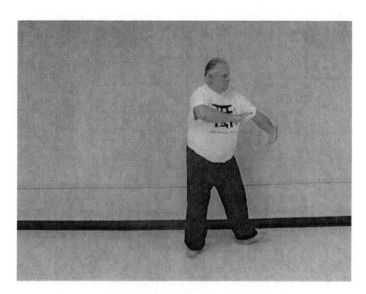

15. Begin Part Horses Mane

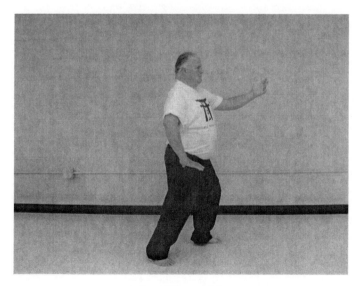

16. Part Horses Mane

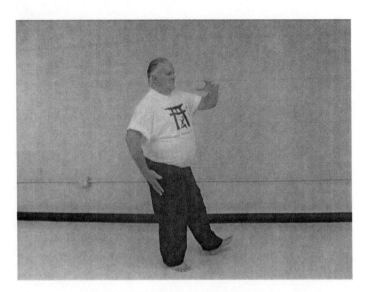

17. Roll Back on Right Leg

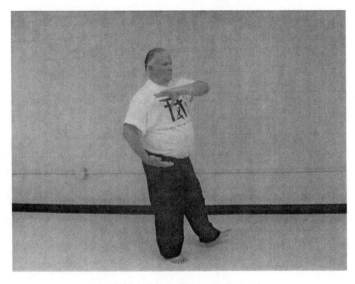

18. Hold the Ball on Right Side

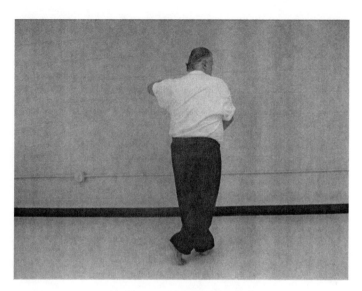

19. Twist 180 Degrees Left

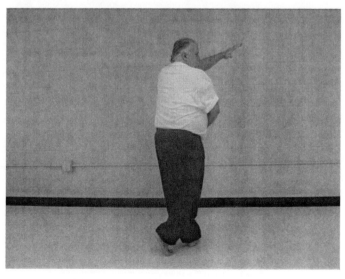

20. Left Hand Moves Past Shoulder

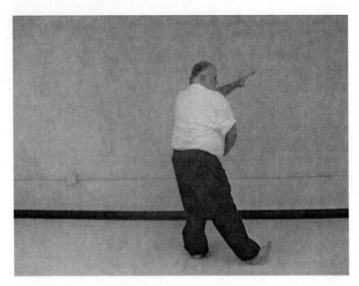

21. Step Foward With Right Leg

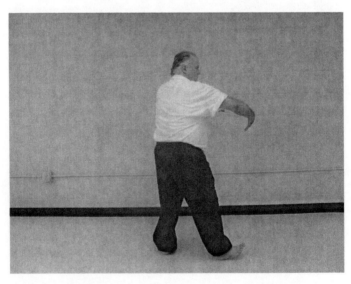

22. Raise Right Hand for Part Horses Mane

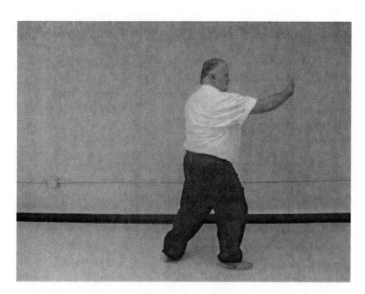

23. Part Horses Mane

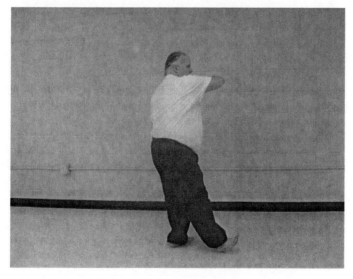

24. Roll Back on Left Foot, Hold the Ball

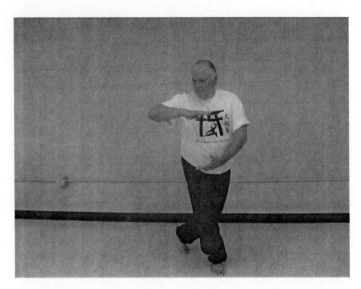

25. Twist 180 Degrees Right

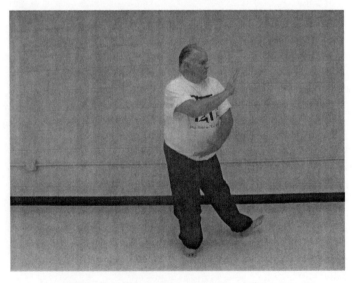

26. Right Hand Foward, Step Foward With Left

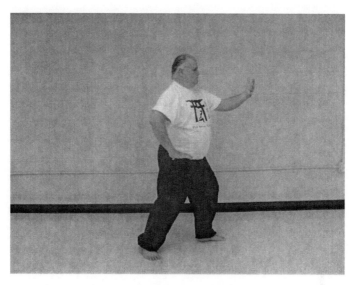

27. Part Horses Mane Completed

TAI CHI LINAGE

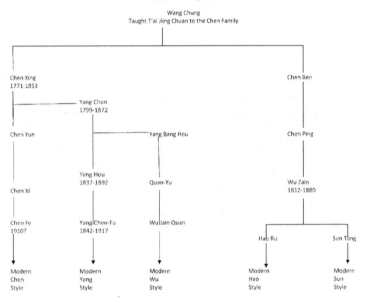

Chen Wang Ting
1391-1458
Founder of T'ai Jiing Chuan

Wang Chung
Taught T'ai Jiing Chuan to the Chen Family

Chen Xing
1771-1853

Chen Ben

Yang Chan
1799-1872

Chen Yun

Yang Bang Hou

Chen Ping

Yang Hou
1837-1892

Quan-Yu

Wu Zain
1812-1880

Chen Xi

Chen Fe
1910?

Yang Chen-Fu
1842-1917

Wu Jain Quan

Hao Ru

Sun Tang

Modern
Chen
Style

Modern
Yang
Style

Modern
Wu
Style

Modern
Hao
Style

Modern
Sun
Style

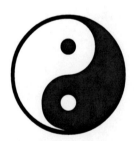

12

PARTING THOUGHTS

To coin a much worn out phrase, "All good things come to an end." Well, I never said I was original. And besides, that phrase is not nearly as old as tai chi, so I guess I am doing pretty well after all.

I truly thank you for reading this book and it would be nice to know that you enjoyed reading it as much as I enjoyed writing it. If you are ever in the Atlanta, Georgia area, look me up. I am not hard to find. I have a website and a FaceBook account. As I was saying, look me up and we will go and have some coffee at my favorite restaurant and enjoy some good conversation. I might even talk about the martial arts, you never can tell. This is the year 2010. If you are reading this book in 2035, never mind. I will either be dead or unable to remember anything about having written a book.

My thoughts drift back to the experience I shared with you about the times when I was a little boy and would go to the movies not caring when the movie started. Back then, as I would leave the theater, I would think to myself, "Wow, it is still daylight out here. It is still Saturday, even though it seems we were at the movies a long time." As we were leaving the theater and walking to the bus stop to catch a ride home, I would often look back and think, "You know, even though I am gone, that movie is still playing back there, but now it is playing for someone else."

Quite by accident, I discovered that is a good analogy for tai chi. Tai chi was in play before I ever came in on it, and long after I am gone, it will still be in play; continuing to unfold for people not even born yet. As a parting thought, I can't help but wonder when I leave, I mean REALLY leave...... you know, like in the hand basket, I just wonder what will happen to tai chi. Everyone knows that things are constantly evolving, and that being the case, in which direction will tai chi follow?

As a parting thought, I can't help but wonder if some day in the future it will become a silly exercise that is added to water aerobics. Will tai chi find its way into the medical industry and tai chi instructors work hand in hand with physical therapists to help people with arthritis and fall prevention? Will tai chi find its way into the school system to teach a Chinese dance to middle school cheerleaders? Will tai chi forms be a part of the Olympics? Will tai chi be someday standardized with specific rules, such as baseball?

These are trends I already see happening as tai chi becomes more and more popular throughout the world and especially throughout the United States.

However, there is a bit of a nightmare going on that should concern you. The nightmare I am talking about is a movement in this country for people to attend a weekend seminar that is usually conducted by a Chinese person from far away and he will pack some auditorium or a hotel ballroom full of people who are willing to part with hundreds of dollars to observe this man for a day or a weekend and at the end of the seminar there is always a group photo taken that you can purchase for about $10.00 and then you are awarded an instructor's certificate.

What is happening within our society is the market is being flooded with "certified instructors" who at its very best are teaching nothing more than over-simplified tai chi. What is happening to tai chi when people are turning out instructors who do not really know what they are doing or why they are doing it?

Are we becoming a society that wants a quick fix for everything, including tai chi instruction? Has tai chi fallen into the category of what I call a "microwave mentality"? Where everything has to happen for us right now, with no patience involved?

I have nothing to gain by insulting anyone who has attended one of these seminars. It is not my intention to insult or belittle anyone. It shows you are willing to learn and you are willing to sacrifice your money and your time to learn a little bit of tai chi. It may even be you are too busy to do anything else but learn a little about tai chi. To coin a street phrase: "a little bit of something is better than a whole lot of nothing".

The problem is not attending a seminar. The problem is attending a seminar for a weekend and believing you are ready to teach tai chi.

What happens here is that a master simplifies moves to teach them quickly. Then the next generation simplifies these moves to make them even easier and within four generations of doing this we have an easy to learn, over-simplified style of tai chi that truly benefits no one in the way it benefitted people 200 years ago.

That is one of the directions I see tai chi going, and I really hope you are wise enough to realize when you have the real thing and when you do not. I also hope you are strong enough and smart enough to oppose these imitation instructors when you see one.

It would be less confusing if they did not call it tai chi. Perhaps, like in math class, you study pre-algebra. Maybe they could call it pre-tai chi.

I am probably worrying too much. Things always have a way of working out for the good, and sooner or later in the cowboy movie the snake oil salesman always gets tarred and feathered.

Another point about modifying or over-simplifying tai chi that I have learned from experience is this: I have seen that people benefit the most when they learn tai chi the same way it was taught hundreds of years ago with no changes except to speak in English. I have had students with M. S., Parkinson 's Disease, Arthritis, Lupus , Cancer, and a host of physical ailments. I even conduct a class made up of special needs adults, some of whom are severely mentally retarded. All these people, as well as a host of others, do quite well learning traditional, non-modified tai chi and always improve on their situation. I am saying this for your benefit. Never think for a minute that you cannot learn tai chi because you have some physical or medical problems. And do not think someone has to simplify it for you.

As I leave, it has been my desire to leave tai chi better than I found it, and I hope you do so as well. I hope you find the best master ever, and you learn the real thing and pass it on to others. Keep it going as it was meant to be, namely, an ancient martial art with Taoist influence.

And if you don't? If you discover tai chi is not for you, that is perfectly all right. Tai chi is not for everybody and if it is not for you, that is nothing to be ashamed of. However, at least stay active in something physical. Continue to learn something new. Never abandon the thrill of learning something new. I know a woman who is 60 years old who runs three miles a day, practices yoga and just recently started back to school learning conversational Spanish at the junior college. She is trim, fit, in perfect health and looks like someone in their late 30's. Her good looks and healthy condition is a direct result of staying physically active and always seeking new things. She can't tell you what's on TV tonight, but she can tell you how fast she ran her last mile. I encourage you to be more like her if you are not already.

One last parting thought: In spite of how magnificent tai chi can be as a health and exercise program, you still need to take good care of yourself. There once was a tai chi master who gained so much weight he could no longer tie his shoes or bring his knee up to his elbow in "The Golden Rooster" posture. He died of complications due to obesity before he turned 50 years old. Another master had an abundant amount of knowledge and martial arts skills only to go to an early grave due to alcohol and drug abuse. Just because you have mastered a martial art does not mean you are perfect. It does not even mean you are balanced. This is a constant endeavor.

Please be wise, stay balanced.

It is hard to end a book about a subject that truly has no end. I have decided to end it with a personal experience.

On October 4, 1996, to my surprise, there was a tea ceremony that ended with the announcement that I was now promoted to the status of Master. And as such, deserved the respect and privileges of any Master who ever lived.

I said to my Master, "Master Haung, I know how to fight, I know the 24 move form, the 48 moves, the 108 moves, I know how to heal, and I know all the pressure points in the body. I even know the Tao Te Ching". And with tears in my eyes, I asked, "What do I do now?" He said, "You start at the beginning."

THE END

BIBLIOGRAPHY/REFERENCES

Tai Chi Classics
Translated by Waysun Liao
Shambhala Publishing

Tai Chi Chuan, The Chinese Way
Foen Tjoeng Lie
Sterling Publishing

Tai Chi Chuan For Health And Self Defense
Master T.T. Liang
Vintage Books

The Tao Of Health, Sex And Longevity
Daniel Reid
Simon & Schuster

Chinese Healing Arts
Translated by John Dudgeon
Edited By William Berk
Unique Publications

Tao Tae Ching
Lao Tsu, Commentary By Ralph Alan Dale
Barnes and Noble

Outline of Thought In Taoism
Ching Hsi-tai
Jen Min Press

Creativity And Taoism
Chang Chung-yuan
The Julian Press, Harper and Row

The Tao Te Ching, Commentary By Ellen M. Chen
Ellen Chen
Paragon House

A complete Guide To Chi Gung
Daniel Reid
Shambhala

A Guide to The I Ching
Carol K. Anthony
Anthony Publishing Company

What Is Taoism? And Other Studies in Chinese Cultural History
Herrlee G. Creel
The University of Chicago Press

The Tao Of Tai Chi Chuan, Way to Rejuvenation
Jou, Tsung Hwa
Edited by Shoshana Shapiro
The Tai Chi Foundation

BIOGRAPHY OF PHIL ROBINSON

- Golden Gloves Boxer 1957 to 1965
- Student of Karate since 1964
- Student of Tai Chi since 1975
- A Master of Korean Karate, Tang Soo Do
- A Master of Yang Tai Chi Chuan Since 1996
- A 4th Degree Black Belt in American Karate
- A Retired Competitive Kick Boxer
- Certified Sabashi Qigong Instructor
- Has been a Martial Artist over 46 years
- Has studied healing, breathing and diet with the Chinese
- Has written two textbooks about Karate
- Has written one textbook about Tai Chi
- A well respected expert on Ancient Weapons
- Has owned three Karate schools
- Has owned six Tai Chi schools

- Co-founder of U.S. Tai Karate
- Founder of The United Tao Association
- Champion and Grand Champion in Tai Chi Forms competition
- A Taoist Disciple since 1993
- A Husband, A Father, A Grandfather

CPSIA information can be obtained at www.ICGtesting.com
Printed in the USA
LVOW11s2324020316

477538LV00001B/7/P